The
Garlic
Book

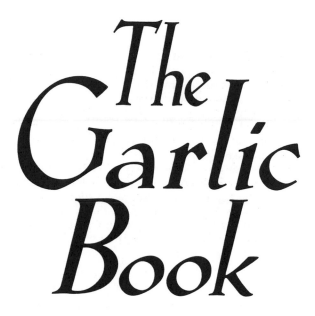

The Garlic Book

NATURE'S POWERFUL HEALER

Stephen Fulder, Ph.D.

Avery Publishing Group

Garden City Park, New York

The therapeutic procedures in this book are based on the training, personal experiences, and research of the author. Because each person and situation are unique, the editor and publisher urge the reader to check with a qualified health professional before using any procedure where there is any question as to its appropriateness.

The publisher does not advocate the use of any particular diet or health program, but believes the information presented in this book should be available to the public.

Because there is always some risk involved, the author and publisher are not responsible for any adverse effects or consequences resulting from the use of any of the suggestions, preparations, or procedures in this book. Please do not use the book if you are unwilling to assume the risk. Feel free to consult with a physician or other qualified health professional. It is a sign of wisdom, not cowardice, to seek a second or third opinion.

Cover design: Bill Gonzalez
In-house editor: Jennifer L. Santo
Printer: Paragon Press, Honesdale, PA

Avery Publishing Group
120 Old Broadway
Garden City Park, NY 11040

Library of Congress Cataloging-in-Publication-Data

Fulder, Stephen.
    The Garlic Book : nature's powerful healer / Stephen Fulder.
      p.   cm.
    Includes bibliographical references and index.
    ISBN 0-89529-786-8
    1. Garlic—Therapeutic use. 2. Heart —Diseases—Diet therapy.
I. Title.
RC684.G37F85 1997
616.1' 206854—dc21   97-7766
                                         CIP

Printed in the United States of America

10 9 8 7 6 5 4 3 2 1

Contents

Acknowledgments

I am most grateful to many experts who have kindly sent me material, especially Dr. Larry Lawson, a pioneer and leading thinker in garlic biomedical research. I thank David Roser for pointing out the need for a popular book that clearly sets out garlic's contribution to the health of our heart and circulation. I also thank the late John Blackwood for his help with editing and for many close and fruitful discussions.

Preface

Most people know garlic only as a tasty addition to food, a major part of many of the world's cuisines. But scientists have recently begun to realize what holistic healers have known for years—that garlic is a valuable natural medicine with many uses. It has long been used to treat infections, ranging from coughs and colds to stomach and skin disorders. Garlic is believed to be especially effective against *Candida*, a yeast infection which is becoming more common in our modern society.

Even more important than its use against infections, garlic has a unique position in the fight against heart disease, a position held by virtually no other remedy. In both these areas, garlic has many advantages over modern drugs. These can be summarized as follows:

- *Garlic works simultaneously on several levels.* Garlic can significantly lower cholesterol and the overall level of fats in the blood, and it is probably as effective as the drugs that are usually used for this purpose. At the same time, it can cause mild reductions in blood pressure. It also thins the blood and prevents clotting or thromboses in the blood vessels. In other words, garlic protects the heart and circulation against the three main causes of atherosclerosis and heart attacks. There are no conventional drugs that act simultaneously at these three critical points. Cholesterol-lowering drugs reduce cholesterol and fats and do have some anticlotting ability, but they do not affect blood pressure. Then, there are drugs that lower blood pressure, but do not affect cholesterol or clotting, and there are mild anti-clotting remedies that do not have the other effects.

- *Garlic is safe.* All drugs (and even, on occasion, some medicinal foods) have side effects. In the case of garlic, however, they are so minimal that the German Federal Health Board declared it to have "no known side effects." A few people do have reactions to fresh garlic—either allergic reactions on the skin while cutting it, or digestive reactions such as nausea and burping, but these effects do not last long, and they are only relevant to fresh garlic. Garlic tablets and other products do not cause these reactions. On the other hand, the drugs used in the management of coronary heart disease, angina, very high cholesterol levels, and other indications of atherosclerosis certainly do have side effects. In the case of blood pressure drugs, for example, side effects range from mild gastric disturbances and mild depression, to asthma and impotence. When it is used against infections, garlic does not cause the side effects some people experience from antibiotics, and there is no danger of the bacteria developing a resistance to garlic, which is sometimes the case when antibiotics are used for long periods of time. Garlic is a harmless medicinal food consumed daily by a large number of people throughout the world. It has been eaten for thousands of years without harm, and with a good deal of benefit. It has, indeed, an astonishing track record for safety.

- *Garlic is a true preventive remedy.* Garlic is a natural remedy which can be incorporated easily into any self-care regimen. It can be taken continuously without the alarming feeling that you have become tied to drugs for the rest of your life. It is the ideal aid if the signs of atherosclerosis are still mild. If, for example, your cholesterol levels are in the grey area above 5.2 mmol/l, or 200 mg/100 ml, but below 6.5 mmol/l, or 250 mg/100 ml, or if your systolic blood pressure is around 150, your medical advisor will be reluctant to start prescribing drugs, which are reserved for more serious cases. Often he or she will do nothing, or very little—perhaps a mention of saturated fat, a warning about smoking, an encouragement to exercise, and a short sermon on peace of mind. Modern medicine is strong on curative prescription but weak on preventive instruction. Yet something must be done to halt the heart disease epidemic. This is where garlic comes into its own—in the intermediate area where prevention is necessary but treatment is not.

- *Garlic is "The People's Medicine."* Garlic is not something that is hard to find and needs experts to explain. It is part of our culture and our human heritage. It is backed by thousands of years of tradition and reliable use. Even in ancient times it was known as "The Peasant's Potion," because simple country folk could cure themselves with it without having to rely on expensive and sophisticated medicine. And talking of expense, garlic can cost no more than the junk food that it should replace. Even in pharmacies, garlic capsules or pills are cheaper than most medicines.

- *Garlic can be a pleasure.* Garlic is more than just a medicine—its flavor forms a key part of the world's cuisine. For those who are attuned to it, garlic provides considerable enrichment to the diet; those who are not can begin by taking capsules or tablets, and may come to appreciate it in time. It fits perfectly into the kind of diet that will help to prevent cardiovascular problems.

This book will provide you with the information you need to make garlic part of your everyday life. The prevention of heart disease is garlic's most important role; this forms the major topic of the book, and will be discussed thoroughly in all its aspects. You will learn how heart disease occurs, and how garlic is beneficial in preventing and controlling it. Suggestions are given on how to include garlic in a heart-healthy diet. Garlic's traditional use as a natural medicine is briefly discussed, and the use of garlic to treat various modern infections is also examined. Finally, detailed information is provided about the various types of garlic products available, and how to incorporate them into a self-care regimen for maximum health.

A well-known saying says it all:
L'ail est sante. Mangez de l'ail.
("Garlic is health. Eat it.")

CHAPTER 1

The Potential of Garlic

Today we find garlic on the shelves of every pharmacy and health food store. In the supermarket there are garlic pills in the health section in addition to the bulbs themselves, in all their glory, among the vegetables. Garlic is given as much prominence in the media as any new drug, and a lot more than almost any other herbal remedy. Major articles on its health benefits have appeared in international newspapers and magazines. A page-long piece in the *New York Times* of July 27, 1994 was headed by a cartoon of a woman in a store reaching for garlic in the vegetable section, under a sign saying "with prescription only!" The article pointed out that garlic sales had reached $100 million a year in the United States. Some 300 million garlic capsules are taken annually in the United Kingdom—in fact, no less than five million Europeans take garlic pills every day.

Even more significantly, the scientific and medical journals, from *Scientific American* to *The Lancet*, have published high-quality research on garlic. In their book, *Garlic: The Science and Therapeutic Applications of* Allium Sativum *and*

Related Species, Dr. Heinrich Koch of Germany and Dr. Larry Lawson of the United States reviewed this research and listed 2,240 scientific papers on the subject of garlic. No one can claim, as they used to, that it is a discarded and useless old wives' tale. But equally, no one can claim today that although garlic may work, there is no scientific backing for its medical effectiveness.

Of course, there is nothing new about garlic's use as a medicine. It is one of the oldest remedies known to man, used without interruption for a wide variety of purposes until a century ago. Only since then, during a relatively short period of time, did it disappear from common use as a medicine, along with most herbs, in favor of synthetic drugs. Now, however, garlic is being rediscovered. We are coming to realize that its benefits are highly relevant to some of the most widespread health problems of our time.

THE MAIN USES OF GARLIC

First and foremost, garlic is a preventive remedy against heart disease. The ancient knowledge of Indian and Eastern medicine states that garlic removes fats from the blood and protects the heart. Traditional herb books and professional herbalists and naturopaths always recommend garlic to those with circulatory problems who are at risk for heart attacks. They say that it opens the blood vessels and thins the blood, and a considerable body of modern, scientific research has confirmed the traditional picture. An excess of fat and cholesterol is one of the major causes of the buildup of arterial blockages, and so of heart disease, heart attacks, and strokes. Garlic lowers the levels of fat and cholesterol in the blood, and it does this as well as, or better than, the modern drugs now used for this purpose.

In addition, studies at some major research centers in the United States have confirmed that garlic does indeed thin the blood by reducing its tendency to clot inside the blood vessels. It does this at quite low doses—less than a clove a day can make a difference that is clearly measurable in the laboratory. Since clots can suddenly block blood vessels, they are one of the main immediate causes of heart attacks, angina, and strokes; garlic may be able to directly reduce the risks of these health catastrophes. In addition, garlic is what is known as a "heating" remedy, according to tradition. We can confirm this ourselves, for we all know how pungent and burning fresh garlic is. But what we may not know is the effect of this warming process on our bodies; it makes us sweat and release poisons from the body, and also reduces blood pressure, both additional advantages in the fight against heart problems.

Thus, garlic offers multiple protection to an extent that no single modern drug is able to provide. It is weaker than many modern heart drugs, although not all. For example, garlic lowers cholesterol to the same extent as fibrate drugs such as bezafibrate, but less than the more powerful cholesterol-lowering agents such as simvastatin. Yet when it is part of a self-care regimen for protecting the heart (involving diet, exercise, and a more relaxed approach to daily life), it can make a real and vital contribution to the prevention of heart disease. And above all, it is safe. It is a food that millions of people include in their daily diet throughout life without any ill effects, and there is no evidence in the scientific literature of any adverse effects from taking garlic as a medicine in normal doses.

The other central use of garlic is in the prevention and treatment of infections. Garlic has been found effective at killing a number of harmful bacteria and fungi. Extensive laboratory tests have shown that, though it is milder and less potent than modern antibiotics, it has a broader range of action than any of them and is, of course, safer. So, garlic can play an important role in the self-treatment of chronic and less immediately severe health problems. These include infections of the mouth, throat, and chest (that is to say, colds, coughs, bronchitis, sinusitis, laryngitis, and so on); infections of the stomach, such as "holiday tummy" and gastroenteritis; infections of the skin, such as athlete's foot or ringworm; and infections of the urogenital area, such as thrush or cystitis. It may be particularly effective against *Candida,* a growing modern problem. For best results, though, garlic should be combined with other methods of self-care.

We should also take into account garlic's qualities as a flavoring and as a nutritional component of the diet, enjoyed today by a large part of the world's population. It is still medically effective when taken in food, though it should be in a significant amount, in the region of a couple of cloves. But what is important, as we shall see, is that garlic must be crushed before use in order to liberate the precious medicinal ingredients. After garlic is crushed, it releases a cascade of effective and strong-smelling substances. The chemistry of these substances will be discussed in a later chapter.

THE POPULARITY OF GARLIC

It is not surprising, then, that in recent years there has been a dramatic, worldwide increase in garlic's medicinal status. Backed by so much scientific research, the message of its significance is clear. Since heart disease is now the major cause of death in developed nations, people have been searching for natural remedies which will help the heart harmlessly. Doctors, too, have shown increasing interest. This is partly because the regular medical drugs that are available to reduce the amount of cholesterol in the blood often have side effects, so doctors have been reluctant to prescribe them too widely. Moreover, since around two-thirds of the adult population of the United States has raised cholesterol levels (that is, above 5.2 mmol/l, or 200 mg/100 ml), the drugs would have to be given to two out of three people. Understandably, most doctors are reluctant to turn the majority of the population into patients.

The natural answer is garlic. When I was giving one of my talks on the radio, the anchorman announced that he had been to see a specialist at a major teaching hospital about his heart. He told the specialist that he was a non-smoker, reasonably fit, and a modest eater, and asked what else he could do to reduce the risk of a heart attack. The official advice was: relax and eat garlic.

This advice has certainly been taken to heart in Germany. After a thorough review of the evidence, the Drugs Commission of the German Health Ministry decided that garlic is a medicine "for assisting in the dietary treatment of raised blood fat levels" and for "preventing age-related deterioration of the circulation." Garlic became, in 1990–1991, the best-selling remedy in German pharmacies. Garlic is not so much a natural part of the German diet as it is in other countries, and many people prefer to take it in the form of tablets and capsules. Its popularity there as a medicine is indeed astonishing. Nearly one million Germans now regularly take garlic products, mostly as a prevention against heart disease. In Japan too, garlic preparations are accepted by the Health Ministry as a means of reducing blood pressure. Garlic appears in the official drug guides (or pharmacopoeiae) of other countries, including Spain and Switzerland, as well.

Similar developments are taking place in the United Kingdom. According to a recent poll, 10 percent of the British population has used garlic or garlic products for medicinal purposes. The British medical authorities have not yet accepted that garlic is effective in circulatory problems. They have, however, acknowledged its other main popular use, that of combating infections. Much of the consumption of garlic products in the United Kingdom occurs for infections of the stomach, throat, mouth, chest, and urogenital area, and in this, too, there is backing from scientific research. The United Kingdom's Ministry of Health allows the product manufacturers to claim that garlic is "an herbal remedy traditionally used for the treatment of the symptoms of common cold and cough" and "an herbal remedy traditionally used for the temporary relief of symptoms of rhinitis and catarrh." This is cautious; however, it does show that the United Kingdom's leading drug experts, though extremely conservative by nature, do recognize garlic's medicinal potential. It is clear that it is a highly popular natural medicine, widely accepted throughout the world and steadily becoming acknowledged by the medical authorities.

FOOD, MEDICINE, OR BOTH?

It might seem strange to you that a food can also be a medicine. Can you really go to your kitchen shelves and find a pharmacy spread out there? Could there really be something to the *New York Times* cartoon of "Prescription Only" vegetables? To anyone with experience of herbs, or to anyone who has lived within the rich cultural tradition of countries like India and China, there is little doubt about the answer. Foods can be medicines and medicines can be foods. There is a great deal of knowledge concerning how to incorporate special foods into the diet so as to prevent and treat a multitude of health problems. Examples that are familiar to us in the West include fiber for digestive problems; oats, barley, and tea to lower cholesterol; vegetables containing beta-carotene to help prevent cancer; olive oil to help prevent heart disease; and so on. In some societies this knowledge is vast, and takes years to learn. I experienced this at first hand in India, where, in traditional families, the mother designs the daily menu to include those foods, vegetables, and spices that are specific for the place, the season, and the weather, and that treat any special vulnerability or health problem within the family.

Spices are on the borderline between food and medicine. It may be hard to visualize those dry old powders in bottles at the back of the kitchen shelves as actual medicines. However, consider for a moment the bombshell to the body locked up in a few grains of cayenne pepper, the anesthetic effect of chewing cloves for a sore tooth, the miraculous way a cup of strong sage tea will clear up a cold and thyme tea a sore throat, and how onion with honey will stop a cough. If anyone has experienced how anise or fennel seeds can treat an upset stomach, how a piece of ginger can get rid of morning sickness, how celery or parsley seed will stop stomach or urinary infections, or how licorice will heal a gastric ulcer, they know something of the power of medicinal foods. It is a knowledge that has generally been lost in the modern world.

Culinary herbs and spices may have distinct advantages as medicines. In the first place they are extremely safe, and unlike many modern drugs, they cannot damage our health while treating our diseases. Second, they are cheap and readily available all over the world. Garlic, for example, is found everywhere and can be many times cheaper than modern cholesterol-lowering drugs. Third, spices can be effective in areas where modern drugs would be strong and unnecessary; many mild, common household health problems, from indigestion to headaches, can be treated by medicinal foods without going to the doctor. Fourth, medicinal foods can prevent disease, whereas there is almost nothing in the modern doctor's medicine chest—apart from vaccines—to strengthen your resistance. Fifth, spices do have some important nutritional benefits; they provide extra vitamins, minerals, and other food factors. Last but not least, they are part of our culture, the true "people's medicine." As people have been doing for thousands of years, herbs and spices, especially garlic, can be included in the natural self-care of many common family health problems, without people having to be constantly dependent on medical professionals.

CHAPTER 2

A Brief History
of Garlic

Mankind and garlic have had a long and passionate relationship. Garlic, in its cultivated form, has needed man to ensure its propagation. But just as much, man has needed garlic to guard his health, well-being, and vigor. This book will deal principally with the present day, with the modern research which has been carried out on garlic and what it can do to help in the current epidemic of heart disease. The situation is urgent, the possibilities dramatic, and the scientific justification and backing far more substantial than most people realize. First, however, to set the stage, we will discuss the details of garlic's past, which is a fascinating one, both as a food and as a medicine.

GARLIC IN ANCIENT TIMES

Dig up the past and you'll find garlic everywhere. Little clay models of garlic bulbs were found in a 6,000 year-old Egyptian burial ground at El Mahasana. The tomb of King

Tutankhamen himself contained six dried bulbs; perhaps they were there to provide him with essential sustenance during his long journey through the afterlife. The Egyptians clearly appreciated garlic, both as an enrichment of the diet and as an important medicine. A 3,500 year-old Egyptian medical text, the Ebers Papyrus, lists twenty-two garlic recipes for problems such as stomach infections, boils, bodily weaknesses, and infected glands.

Garlic was the fare of ancient kings, and was also relied on for taste, strength, and nourishment by the common folk. The Jews in the wilderness, according to the Bible (Numbers 11:4–6), became so bored with their monotonous diet of manna that they longed for the garlicky food of Egypt, even though they had eaten it as slaves. The ancient Greeks loved their garlic, and Aristotle recommended it as a tonic. The Romans, too, were typically Mediterranean in their appreciation of garlic. Virgil praised its restorative power for reapers during the long, hot harvest. Roman legions planted it wherever they were stationed, in vegetable plots beyond the walls of their camps. They believed that it made them fighting fit and more aggressive. In fact, the Roman wish, "May you not eat garlic" was the equivalent of saying, "May you not be drafted."

Throughout history, garlic has been valued as a medicine as well as a food. Hippocrates, who lived on the Greek island of Kos and is considered the forefather of modern medicine, praised garlic for driving out excess water from the body, settling upset stomachs, and curing infections and inflammations. This is one of his remedies for an infected lung: "And if you recognize the signs of suppuration, the sick man, for his evening meal and before he goes to bed, should eat raw garlic in great quantity and should drink a noble and pure wine. If by this means the pus erupts, so much the better."

Dioscorides, the Roman physician whose understanding of plants has been the inspiration of herbalists right up to the present day, had this to say about it: "Garlic ... makes the voice clear and soothes continuous coughing when eaten raw or boiled. Boiled with oregano, it kills lice and bed bugs. It clears the arteries. Burnt and mixed with honey, it is an ointment for bloodshot eyes; it also helps baldness. Together with salt and oil, it heals eczema. Together with honey, it heals white spots, herpetic eruptions, liver spots, leprosy, and scurvy. Boiled with pinewood and incense, it soothes tooth-ache when the solution is kept in the mouth. Garlic with fig leaves and cumin is a plaster against the biting of the shrew-mouse. . . . A mush from crushed garlic and black olives is a diuretic. It is helpful in dropsy."

Galen, one of the true fathers of medicine, called it the "countryman's cure-all" (*theriacum rusticorum*) and Gaius Pliny, the greatest natural historian of ancient times, compiled an astonishing list of up to fifty disorders that garlic would cure. Pliny died observing the eruption of Vesuvius which buried Pompeii—in whose ashes garlic was, of course, found preserved.

GARLIC IN MEDIEVAL TIMES

The Romans presumably brought garlic with them to England, where it became valued as a flavoring for goose. Throughout medieval and Renaissance Europe, it was a familiar part of life, and its smell was a part of its fun. A contemporary source mentions how Henry IV of France, who ruled from 1589 to 1610, chewed garlic and had "a breath that would fell an ox at twenty paces." At the same time, its health-giving qualities were praised by all the leading herbalists. By their theory of elements and humors, garlic was regarded as very "heating and drying," and was therefore used to combat "moist" and "cold" diseases, including catarrh and boils, various stubborn infections, and sluggish circulation of the blood. According to Queen Elizabeth's herbalist, William Turner, it "maketh subtill the nourishment and the blood," implying that it cleared blockages in both. This statement is, of course, of great interest to us today.

GARLIC AND CLASS DISTINCTIONS

By around 1600 a prejudice against garlic's pungency began to develop in northern, Protestant Europe. Garlic became one of the signs of class distinction; it was now regarded as the food of rustics and peasants, and not suited to the refined palates of the upper classes. This is shown in Shakespeare's *Measure for Measure,* Act III, Scene ii, where Lucio says of the Duke that he would "mouth with a beggar though she smell brown bread and garlic." In 1699, in his book on salads, the famous diarist John Evelyn wrote of garlic, "We absolutely forbid it entrance into our salleting by reason of its intolerable rankness." Spaniards, Italians, and French people might eat it, so might countrymen—especially if they lived in damp places—and sailors, but it was definitely beneath the dignity of English ladies and gentlemen. During the nineteenth century this distaste was well expressed by the culinary and domestic "guru" Mrs. Beeton. As she wrote in her *Book of Household Management,* "The smell of this plant is generally considered offensive. . . . It was in greater repute with our ancestors than it is with ourselves, although it is still used as a seasoning or herb."

The dislike spread with the Anglo-Saxons to the United States, where surveys conducted on the subject of tastes always seem to find garlic is the most unpopular flavor of all, along with olive oil. (At the top of the list are banana, chocolate, and strawberries.) This prejudice is, in part, still with us and must be taken seriously. How did it come about? To judge by the various cutting remarks in Shakespeare and other sources, it arose because aristocratic people began to express their refinement through a new, starched cleanliness. Pungent smells became the province of the poor; for the rich it was all lavender and roses. As the process continued, bland tastes and odors became associated with self-discipline, primness, and restraint. Garlic was associated with the forbidden passions indulged in by Mediterranean peoples, and with the repellent grubbiness of the working classes.

Now, however, a change is coming about. Today the health-conscious middle and upper classes eat garlic, along with brown, whole wheat bread and other natural foods. The old, bland, inoffensive cooking is seen as inhibited and unhealthy, as well as unnecessary. The return to a natural lifestyle is being accompanied by an acceptance of natural smells.

GARLIC AS A TRADITIONAL MEDICINE

Let us look more closely at garlic as a traditional medicine. The language and practices of the old herbals can seem picturesque and confusing if one does not know how to extract the essential truth and common sense contained in them. This is particularly the case with garlic, as it appears to have such a bewildering array of uses. Nevertheless, once these are summarized rationally and consistently, a familiar picture emerges.

The Use of Garlic Against Infections

Garlic was especially recommended by herbalists in infections of the stomach (such as dysentery), mouth, throat (such as sore throat, coughs, and catarrh), ears, and skin. It was used both internally and externally for boils, spots, carbuncles, and ulcers. During the First World War it was extensively used by both sides to treat infected wounds. In the British trenches, sterilized sphagnum moss containing garlic juice was generally placed over the injury. Reports from that time describe it as a successful front-line protection against gangrene. It was also used in the trenches against dysentery, a practice continued during the Second World War by the countries of Eastern Europe.

Garlic has been used against some very ugly infections indeed. Very large doses, or "saturation doses," were used, with some effectiveness, to treat tuberculosis and leprosy, something which still continues in remote areas of the world. It was also used against cholera and typhoid with considerable success, according to medical and popular records. Dr. Albert Schweitzer used it in this way in Africa. Even the plague, while not cured by garlic, may have been deterred by it; French priests who attended the bedsides of victims in eighteenth-century London remained healthy, while the non-garlic-eating English priests succumbed.

The Use of Garlic for Bites, Stings, and Poisons

Garlic is widely spoken of as the foremost first aid remedy against the assaults of the more unpleasant side of the animal kingdom. Aristotle recommended it for the bites of mad dogs, and Mohammed for scorpion stings; the author can personally vouch for the latter in the case of a certain common, nonlethal, but unpleasant Middle Eastern scorpion. Greek and Roman herbalists called it an antidote to snakebite, and told how farmers would carry it with them in the fields as an emergency remedy. There were other antitoxic effects, the most famous being its ability to deal with a hangover. In France, the recommended "morning after" cure was a soup made of onions and garlic.

The Use of Garlic for the Circulation

Garlic clears the arteries, said Dioscorides, as did William Turner after him, and it was consistently used to cure "blockages" or "stiffness" of the blood system. The relatively common disease known as "dropsy," in which part or all of the body swelled up and became waterlogged, arose from poor circulation. Today, we know this condition as edema. Early English doctors talk of garlic's heat as "boiling away the fluid" of dropsy, and garlic became the principal treatment for this. In Asian—especially Indian—medicine, garlic was specifically used to remove fat from the blood and dry out excess moisture from the body. (By the same token, they noted that it reduced the amount of milk produced by breast-feeding mothers, and they advised them to be careful of their consumption). Charaka, the traditional father of Indian medicine, stated that garlic maintains the fluidity of the blood and strengthens the heart, and traditional Indian physicians nowadays rely on garlic and onion "lasona" therapy to prevent heart disease.

Other Miscellaneous Uses

Garlic was used to treat tumors and growths on the skin, and also scurvy. Rheumatism and piles are also mentioned. Some of these various uses probably relied on garlic's ability to heat the body and cause sweating, and therefore, cleansing. Garlic was used to control infestations of intestinal worms in people and animals. This is still an extremely important effect in poorer parts of the world. It is also supposed to deter fleas and lice from biting.

The traditional explanation of how garlic "maketh subtill the blood" tells us that the old herbalists really understood something of how it achieves this important effect. It resulted, they said, from garlic's heating and drying properties, which removed water from the body and opened "cold," atrophied, and blocked blood vessels. Today, of course, we would call the condition of these blocked vessels atherosclerosis, and speak of degenerative diseases of the circulation, which means much the same thing. The use of garlic in circulatory problems will be the main theme of this book. Here we see that it has an ancient precedent.

CHAPTER 3

Getting To Know Garlic

Garlic's botanical name is *Allium sativum;* this means that it belongs to the Allium group of plants, in which there are some 600 species. These include onions, chives, leeks, wild garlic (ransoms), shallots, rakkyo, kurrat, and various other ornamental and wild species. They all belong to the lily family. Garlic, like most of the members of this family, has spear-like leaves, about 6 inches (15 cm) long. (Its English name comes from this; it is the Anglo-Saxon *garleac,* or spear-plant.) These leaves originate from the fleshy base of the stem, which is the head (or bulb) of garlic. A bunch of thin roots emerge from the bottom of the head like a beard. The head of garlic consists of eight to twenty cloves clustered together, covered by a thin papery skin which may be white or mauve-grey. The stem of garlic sometimes produces purple-white flowers. These are not fertile, and unlike the wild form, cultivated garlic cannot be grown from seed.

Garlic is grown from its own clove. This should be placed, tip uppermost, 2 inches (5 cm) under the soil. The

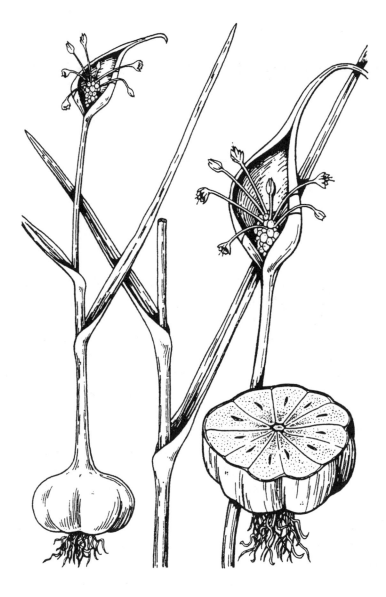

Left: Mature, flowering garlic plant.
Right: Cross-section of garlic bulb, showing cloves.

best time to plant garlic is at the end of November. It requires a rich soil, but it is not very fussy about the weather. Garlic can be planted anywhere from the cold of the Catskills to the dry heat of New Mexico. The plant will emerge in late winter, grow throughout the spring, and be ready for harvest in the summer. The fleshy substance of the clove provides the young shoot with food while it is developing, and also contains the unique substances that provide us humans with flavoring and medicine.

A great deal of garlic is grown and consumed in the world, much of it in ready-made flavorings. According to United Nations trade statistics, enough garlic is grown to give each member of the human race half a clove a day. China is the biggest producer, followed by India, Spain, and various Mediterranean countries. The United States alone consumed 500 million pounds of garlic in 1994, enough to give each person in the country about three-quarters of a clove every day. This is quite a lot of garlic for a country that views garlic as the most hated smell among foods. Ninety percent of America's garlic is grown at home, much of it in Gilroy, California, the "garlic capital of America." It is said that in the harvest season, the smell can be detected many miles away. Gilroy hosts an annual garlic celebration at which a growing number of garlic aficionados can enjoy themselves.

GARLIC'S SECRET: SULFUR

Garlic contains some remarkably strong and unique substances. What is it that can keep the arteries open; kill bacteria, yeasts, and fungi; heat the body and drive out poisons; and even kill insects, all in relatively small dosages and without side effects? The key to garlic's potency is found in one element: sulfur. Even more than the other alliums, garlic has the ability to accumulate some very unusual sulfur compounds. After some fifty years of research involving leading natural product chemists, including Professor Artur Vitaanen, a Nobel prizewinner, the main secrets of garlic's strength were revealed. Like all scientific discoveries, it began with a puzzle. How is it that a clove of garlic, when intact, has no smell or taste, but when it is crushed or cut, the strong smell and typical garlic taste are immediately created? (This only works when the garlic is fresh. If you boil a clove of garlic, it completely loses the ability to generate that garlic power—it tastes just like a vegetable. Try it!)

The answer was found in 1944 by scientists working for the Winthrop Chemical Company in the United States. They found that garlic is rich in a substance called *alliin*, which is a special sulfur-containing version of an amino acid. The amino acids are the building blocks from which proteins are constructed. Alliin has almost no smell or taste. However, as soon as garlic is crushed or chopped, alliin mixes inside the garlic tissues with an enzyme (a biological catalyst) called *allinase;* this sets off a chemical reaction that quickly changes the alliin into another compound called *allicin.* This smells strongly, has a pungent, fiery taste, and is very active, both as a chemical and as a medicine. It is the substance that burns the tongue when you bite into a fresh clove of garlic. The burning sensation of allicin gives us an idea of what all those strange compounds are doing in the garlic bulb in the first place—they are the garlic's own chemical weapon against insects. You can imagine the explosion of allicin that would meet a marauding pest foolish enough to take a bite out of a garlic bulb!

After crushing, garlic becomes a veritable witches' brew of substances, for allicin is highly reactive. In fact, it is so reactive that it changes of its own accord into a range of other sulfur compounds, mainly sulfides. These have a strong, heavy aroma—the typical smell of garlic—giving rise to its affectionate European slang name, "the Stinking Rose." These sulfides are made rapidly from the original allicin when garlic is heated after crushing, as in cooking. They are made more slowly if the crushed garlic is left standing, even in the refrigerator. After a few days, garlic does not contain any of the original allicin—it has all been converted into sulfides. The main sulfide is called *diallyl disulfide,* but there are many others. The sulfides are oily; they are the main active constituents of the garlic oil capsules that you can purchase in health stores.

After much debate over the years, it has now been conclusively proved that allicin is the main active medicinal compound in garlic. It has been known for over fifty years that if you take allicin out of garlic and use it in simple laboratory tests to kill bacteria and fungi, it will do so as well as the whole garlic. But if garlic is boiled or treated so there is no allicin, it actually helps the growth of bacteria, rather than preventing it. This has been confirmed many times, and even the Nobel prizewinner Artur Vitaanen has shown that allicin must be present for garlic to work. In studies at the Department of Microbiology at the University of Indiana, many garlic compounds were checked to see how they rated as natural antibiotics. Only allicin, or the daughter compounds created when allicin breaks down, were effective.

A similar picture exists in relation to the effect of garlic on the circulation. Virtually all of the thirty-five clinical studies carried out to date on garlic and the circulation used fresh, dried, or distilled garlic containing allicin and/or its daughter compounds. A team of researchers at the U.S. Department of Agriculture laboratories in Madison, Wisconsin, have tested many different extracts of garlic for their ability to help lower cholesterol levels. Only those extracts that contained or had contained allicin were effective. We should remember that allicin quickly breaks down into sulfides and garlic oil, and these are also effective. When we talk about "allicin," we mean allicin and/or all its end products. Allicin must be present, or, like the yeast that makes the bread rise but is then destroyed in baking, must have been present, even if it has been transformed. For that reason, when assessing garlic products, experts often talk about "allicin yield" rather than "allicin content."

Scientists are also now beginning to have some idea of what happens to garlic's powerful chemicals once they enter the body. If you eat crushed garlic or garlic powder, you will be taking in a combination of allicin and the precursor substances, especially alliin, leftovers that have not yet been converted to the active allicin compound. In the intestine, the leftover alliin is probably all converted to allicin. The allicin begins to pass through the walls of the digestive tract into the body. As it does so, the unstable allicin is converted to sulfides and similar compounds called mercaptans, which are the compounds that appear to be active inside the body. Within a few hours, the sulfur compounds are excreted in the urine.

THE GARLIC GALAXY

Garlic, like all natural herbal remedies, contains a galaxy of chemical substances, many of which affect our bodies. The allicin is the most important substance in garlic in terms of both amount and medicinal power. But there are, of course, many others. One interesting group, researched by Professor Erick Block of the State University of New York at Albany, includes ajoene and vinyl dithiins. These are created when garlic is fried or macerated in oil, or in the laboratory when it is crushed and mixed with alcohol. They are very powerful anticlotting substances. There are also small quantities of compounds based on the amino acid cysteine. Garlic is related to onion, and indeed, not only does garlic contain substances that taste and smell like onion (such as propenyl disulfide), but onion creates similar substances to allicin when it is cut or crushed, and it is these that make you cry.

The allicin constitutes from 0.3 to 1 percent of the weight of garlic, although it makes up in power what it lacks in quantity. The amounts of allicin, and of the active sulfur compounds, can vary extensively in different garlic bulbs grown in different fields, different countries, and different ways. For example, Chinese garlic is quite rich in active ingredients, as is garlic that is grown organically (in soil that has not been chemically treated). Research suggests that some microorganisms in the soil are important in making sulfur compounds from the earth available to the hungry roots of the garlic plant. And, of course, a bit of sulfur added to the soil will help them along.

Garlic is 60 percent water, and each clove, which may weigh from 2 to 5 grams (about one-eighth of an ounce), contains approximately one gram of carbohydrates, 0.2 grams of protein, a little fat, and small amounts of B complex vitamins, vitamins C and E, and the antioxidant mineral selenium. Though garlic is the richest source of selenium among the edible plants, very little garlic is eaten, compared, for example, to fish (which is also high in selenium), so the actual amount of this valuable mineral that garlic contributes to the diet is minimal. The same can be said for the other vitamins and nutrients in garlic.

Garlic, with its sulfurous nature, is clearly both fierce and friendly. There is an ancient legend to that effect. Having brought about the Fall of Man, Satan stepped from the Garden of Eden; where his right foot first rested, the onion plant sprang up, and where his left foot met the ground, there grew garlic. This dual quality of cursing and blessing typifies garlic's pungent power. Let us see how we can make the best use of it.

CHAPTER 4

Understanding
Heart Disease

The present day has opened a new chapter in the long history of garlic as a medicinal remedy. As we have seen, the herbalists of the past knew something of garlic's beneficial effect on the circulation, though they were more concerned with its anti-infective power, since they didn't suffer from heart disease as we do today. Now we know a great deal more, and that knowledge has become extremely important to us. For one of our greatest failings in the field of health is our inability to control diseases of the heart and circulation, which now claim more lives than any other single cause. We need to understand, then, how heart disease arises and how garlic can be used, together with other precautions, to keep it in check.

THE MODERN EPIDEMIC

The first thing to realize is how much heart disease is a problem of our own making. It is a modern problem that arises from two main general causes. The first is that almost all of us now live to an age at which diseases which build up over a period of time are able to show themselves. Consider the fact that a hundred years ago, three-quarters of the people of Europe would not have reached their seventieth birthdays. Today, only one in three fail to make it. The big killers used to be the infectious diseases, such as tuberculosis, diphtheria, venereal disease, cholera, and septicemia. After these were subdued, largely through developments in public health and sanitation, life expectancy increased considerably. However, the victory was only partial. The door was then left open for new kinds of diseases—the degenerative conditions of mid- and later life, especially cancer and circulatory diseases. The chances of suffering from these diseases are as great as they ever were, if not more so; because of this, a forty-year-old man today is no more likely to reach old age than was a forty-year-old man a hundred years ago. Heart disease and cancer together cause four out of every five deaths in middle age. Heart disease alone causes one out of two deaths. Although there has been an improvement in this trend in America compared with northern Europe, brought about because of reduced smoking and more exercising (the "fitness revolution"), heart disease is still a major cause of adult mortality.

HOW CIRCULATORY PROBLEMS DEVELOP

In order to understand how garlic can help the circulation, we should consider how circulatory problems occur. The same basic process underlies most circulatory disorders. It begins with the gradual blocking or furring-up of the arteries. Like a drain that slowly becomes blocked by accumulating layers of waste, the arteries collect streaks and lumps of fat on their inside surfaces. This occurs especially at certain sites, for example, at the places where the blood vessels divide and branch.

This buildup is the palpable sign—the tip of the iceberg—of an invisible process occurring all the time. It may start with slight damage to the artery lining, which precipitates the first stage of the body's repair mechanism. Small cell pieces called *platelets* (which are the advance guard of the clotting process) arrive and stick to the damaged area; these act as flags and attract other cells involved in clotting. Globules of cholesterol, always present in the bloodstream, join the platelets and form a spot or clot on the arterial lining. House-cleaning, scavenger cells migrate to the area. They attempt to clean up by removing the clot, but in doing so they become so engorged with the excessive amounts of cholesterol present that they remain as fatty lumps; they are like a vacuum cleaner which becomes so overstuffed that it breaks down. More and more cholesterol accumulates at the site, and the result is a fatty deposit or plaque. Since antioxidants such as vitamins C and E can help to slow this process, it is now thought that the oxidation, or deterioration, of fats and cholesterol is partly to blame for cholesterol's unwanted stickiness. In time, the deposits so swell the interior surfaces of the blood vessels that the passageway becomes partially blocked. The blockage is called a sclerosis, and the process of blockage is known as *atherosclerosis.*

Atherosclerosis increases with age and time, and exists to some degree in all adults. When it is severe, it can itself trigger the blood-clotting mechanism normally reserved for sealing up breaks, since the body regards the narrowed vessels themselves as damaged and in need of repair. A clot which forms inside a vessel like this is called a *thrombosis.* The vessels that seem to be most at risk for thromboses are those that bring the blood to the hardest-working muscle in the whole body, the heart. These are called the coronary vessels; a clot that dams up these vessels is therefore called a coronary thrombosis. It stops blood from reaching the heart, causing chest pain, angina, or, if more severe, a heart attack.

Other blood vessels that are particularly vulnerable are those in the brain; if a thrombosis occurs here, it can lead to a stroke. Heart attack and stroke are the most common results of atherosclerosis. However, there can be other results, such as an increase in blood pressure.

THE INSIDE INVESTIGATION

We all might benefit from understanding the origins of atherosclerosis and the factors that will make the situation worse or better. We need to discover methods that will reduce the risk of heart attacks and other serious conditions. The questions we must ask are: Can atherosclerosis be stopped and reversed? If so, what kinds of remedies and preventive methods can be used? How genuinely reliable and effective are they?

The very first indications of the causes of the process of atherosclerosis were obtained from a study not of the sick but of the healthy. Ever since 1948, thousands of inhabitants of the town of Framingham, Massachusetts, have been giving a detailed picture of their lifestyle to investigators from the U.S. National Heart, Lung, and Blood Institute. The researchers also checked these people at regular yearly intervals for heart disease. Gradually, the picture emerged that those most likely to suffer from heart disease were also more likely to be eating a lot of animal fat, to be smoking cigarettes, and to have raised blood pressure.

At first, neither the U.S. government health authorities nor health scientists in general took much notice of these findings. The prevailing view at that time was that diseases were caused by outside agencies like bacteria, and not by the way we lived. Over the last thirty years or so, however, evidence has accumulated to the contrary. It became clear that those of the world's peoples who still live in the traditional way, without packaged, processed foods and the stress and toxicity of modern life, such as the Australian aborigines and the Masai of Africa, never suffer from heart disease, unless they began to live in the modern way. It emerged, as the natural practitioners had said all along, that heart disease was the result of a variety of separate causes, and that these could be summed up in two words: living unnaturally.

Enormous research projects, studying the life habits of hundreds of thousands of people, have been carried out at a cost of millions of dollars. Various specific factors were identified as the main causes of heart disease: a high proportion of animal fats in the diet; smoking; high blood pressure; diabetes and other problems with sugar metabolism; lack of fitness and aerobic exercise; being overweight; and stress. Some specific dietary factors are also coming to light, such as deficiencies of certain vitamins and minerals (particularly magnesium, C, E, and B complex), which naturopaths have always known about.

THE STRESS FACTOR

Stress is a profound problem. Researchers found that people who were tense, over-conscientious, ambitious, and under strain had a much higher chance of incurring heart attacks, even if they did not indulge themselves in doughnuts and hamburgers. Recently, psychologists have gone a little deeper and found that those people who are tense and cannot fully relax are often disconnected from themselves, perhaps from guilt or denial, and this leads to stress. The anxieties, loneliness, distance within the family and the society, and lack of warmth in daily life are deep cultural disturbances of modern man, and they have physical as well as emotional effects. This psychological dimension, along with other factors such as food quality and lack of exercise, is seen as one of the reasons why our ancestors were not bedeviled by heart disease, despite a fat-laden diet.

REACHING A VERDICT ON CHOLESTEROL

Cholesterol is a type of fat needed by the body as the starting point in the manufacture of a variety of important materials, particularly hormones. Some cholesterol is obtained from the diet, but most is made by the liver. If the body is under continuous stress, it needs more stress hormones such as corticosteroid; the liver makes large amounts of cholesterol so that there is plenty of raw material available for the manufacture of these hormones. The amount of cholesterol in the blood is influenced by several factors:

- The amount of cholesterol in the diet.

- The consumption of saturated fats (the types of fat found in all animal and dairy products), which encourages the liver to make more cholesterol.

- Stress and the production of adrenaline (for example, the blood of race-car drivers after a race becomes milky with fat droplets).

- Obesity (large amounts of fat stored up in the body).

- Diabetes.

- A lack of fiber in the diet.

- Heredity—some people have a tendency to have higher levels of cholesterol than normal.

- Being physically unfit—exercise can burn up excessive fats and cholesterol.

The amount of cholesterol in the blood is closely linked to atherosclerosis and heart attacks. This can be clearly seen in laboratory studies in which animals are given excessive amounts of cholesterol, but also by comparing different human populations. For example, the highest level of cholesterol in the world used to occur in the males of East Finland at 6.9 millimols to every liter (mmol/l), or 265 milligrams to every 100 milliliters (mg/ml), of blood. The heart attack rate there was fourteen times greater than the place with the lowest level, Japan, which had an average of 4.1 mmol/l, or 160 mg/100 ml. Proportionally, cholesterol levels have a very large influence on heart disease: a 10 percent reduction in cholesterol brings down the incidence of disease by 20 percent.

In America, the average blood cholesterol level is now 205 mg/100 ml. It has gone down slightly in the last thirty years, from 220 mg/100 ml. This is thought to be because of changes in diet, especially the reduction in the consumption of animal fat. Heart attacks have been reduced by one-third, and the average life span has increased by three years. It is supposed that this represents improvements in fitness and in medicine as well as changes in food.

In the United Kingdom, there has been very little change in diet, lifestyle, fitness, cholesterol levels, or heart attack rates. Women before menopause are much less likely to get heart attacks and heart disease than men of the same age, but after menopause the risk for women increases, and above the age of 65 it is nearly the same as the risk for men. Estrogen therapy during menopause can significantly reduce the risk of heart disease, although at the cost of a slightly increased risk of breast cancer. Life expectancy in the United Kingdom is lower than it is in the United States, and Scotland, in particular, has the unenviable reputation of being the country with the highest level of heart disease in the world. Thus, all the indicators now point to raised cholesterol levels as one of the main causes of heart disease. Indeed, the National Institutes of Health states that cholesterol is not only a risk factor, it is actually a central cause of the problem.

The World Health Organization has looked at cholesterol levels worldwide and has stated that, for cardiac health, they should be at a maximum of 5.2 mmol/l, or 200 mg/100 ml. Unfortunately, two-thirds of the adult population of modern, post-industrial countries are above this figure. This is a serious situation. Some medical authorities suggest that all such people should be given cholesterol-lowering drugs, but this is surely absurd. It would make the majority of adults in these countries feel like patients, greatly enrich certain drug companies at everyone's expense, and open a Pandora's box of possible side effects. Worst of all, it would divert effort away from taking the natural preventive measures that are within everyone's reach.

LDL AND HDL

Before we can understand how to improve cholesterol levels, we must deepen our knowledge of how cholesterol is handled within the body. It does not simply float around in oily drops. Each tiny droplet is contained within a bag of protein called *lipoprotein*, which makes it soluble in the blood. There are several types of cholesterol bags, but the ones that concern us here are called LDL (low-density lipoprotein) and HDL (high-density lipoprotein). Between them, these carry 90 percent of the cholesterol in the blood.

The liver makes cholesterol and sends it out to the fat stores, fatty tissues located throughout the body. There some is taken up, and the rest circulates freely in the blood in the form of LDL. The cells of the body all need small amounts of cholesterol. They take in some of the LDL, remove its cholesterol, and leave the rest of the LDL free. The more cholesterol that enters the bloodstream, the sooner the cells are satisfied, and the more LDL remains in the blood. LDL is known as "bad" cholesterol, and it is the most abundant. It is the one which is taken up by the arteries to create the fatty lumps which cause atherosclerosis. When cholesterol levels are measured, most is present in the form of LDL, so LDL levels are in fact more directly related to the risk of heart attack than the level of cholesterol overall. Saturated fats, excess cholesterol in the diet, and smoking all increase LDL.

High-density lipoprotein (HDL), on the other hand, may actually provide protection against heart attacks. It has now been found that people with high levels of HDL are protected from heart disease even if their overall cholesterol is high. In the Framingham study mentioned earlier, the risk of heart attack was 70 percent higher in those men with HDL less than 52 mg/100 ml, compared to those with more HDL. In women it seemed to make even more of a difference; those whose HDL was less than 46 mg/100 ml were six times more likely to have a heart attack than those with HDL levels above 67 mg/100 ml. HDL seems to act as a kind of house-cleaner, collecting the cholesterol from the walls of the arteries and returning it to circulation. For this reason, the HDL/LDL ratio is very often used as a measure of cardiovascular risk: the higher it is, the better.

CLOTTING AND COAGULATION

As we have seen, a heart attack or stroke is precipitated by a clot which forms in a blood vessel. This occurs when the clotting mechanism is triggered by the presence of a fatty area rather than, as is usual, by a break or wound. The clotting mechanism is a complex cascade of actions and reactions. It originates with sticky cell fragments called platelets, which circulate in the blood. As soon as platelets meet the rough edge of a wound or other damage, they clump together. At the same time, they release an agent which converts a blood protein, *fibrinogen,* to a fibrous material called *fibrin.* The fibrin forms a mesh over the area in which the blood solidifies, forming the clot.

However, there must be an opposite process which puts a brake on the clotting, otherwise it would continue and block the blood system every time it repaired a cut. This de-clotting, or breaking of the fibrin threads, is called *fibrinolysis,* and when it occurs inside the blood vessels, it prevents the building up of clots. The balance between fibrin formation and fibrinolysis affects the rate at which clotting takes place. A clot normally forms within several minutes. If there is more fibrin being made, it tends to form more quickly. More fibrinolysis, on the other hand, delays clotting, removes unwanted clots, and generally thins the blood. Clearly, it is very important to have this mechanism in good shape in order to prevent thromboses in the furred-up arteries.

Raised LDL cholesterol levels increase fibrin and clot formation and reduce fibrinolysis. Adrenaline, the hormone poured into the blood during stress, also speeds up clotting, and this adds to the chances of a heart attack in those under permanent psychological stress. Tobacco smoke, saturated fats, and lack of exercise have the same effect. On the other hand, diets with the right kinds of fats can promote the fibrinolytic, clot-dissolving activity.

There is a further important dimension to the clotting process. This is the prostaglandin system, the "local messenger service" situated in the walls of the arteries. It dispatches substances which either promote the clumping of platelets and blood clotting (the messenger in this case is a prostaglandin called thromboxane A2) or prevent clumping, reduce clotting, and open blood vessels (achieved by prostacyclin). Since these chemical messengers are also made from the raw material of the fats we eat, we can promote the prostacyclin, clot-preventing system by dietary means.

For example, fish and fish oil are kind to the circulation. Fish oil, in particular, contains a substance called EPA (eicosapentaenoic acid). Our ancestors used to get EPA from wild animals. The flesh of domestic animals does not contain it, so it is present in our diet only in fish. The man who discovered the health benefits of fish oil was Dr. Hugh Sinclair, a nutritional expert from Oxford. In the early 1980s, he went to live with the Eskimos to find out why they have so little heart disease despite a very high-fat diet. He tested their diet, which consists exclusively of fish, and lived on this diet himself. The types of fats in his own bloodstream greatly improved, but he also suffered from nosebleeds and spontaneous wounds because of a reduction in clotting. However, we need not go as far as he did. EPA-rich, natural fish oil supplements have now become a very popular and medically approved method of reducing cholesterol in the blood and preventing unwanted clotting.

THE REMEDY IN THE DIET

Hundreds of studies have demonstrated that animal fats have the unfortunate result of increasing cholesterol, LDL, and blood clotting. This is now well accepted. However, that is not all; the total fat content of the diet contributes to the problem and should be decreased. In Japan—which has the lowest heart disease level of all developed countries—dietary fat makes up about twelve percent of the total intake, whereas in the United Kingdom, the percentage is three times as high.

At birth, a human baby has some 1.3 mmol of LDL cholesterol per liter of blood, or 50 mg/100 ml, and this is the level at which the system is in balance. But in Western countries, the normal adult LDL level is 3.2 mmol/l, or 125 mg/100 ml. It is possible to reduce LDL back to its original level. It has been found that a pure vegan diet, with no dairy products, eggs, or meat, will achieve this. Though few will be able to reach this goal, vegetarians as a whole have much less LDL, together with more HDL and, of course, a lower likelihood of cardiovascular problems.

To study the effects of a vegetarian diet on circulatory health, one needs to compare two groups who live rather similarly, except that some eat meat and some do not. The Seventh-day Adventists are such a group. A study of 24,000 nonsmoking Seventh-day Adventists, done in Holland in 1983, compared those who were vegetarians with those who were not, and found that the meat-eaters were three times more likely to incur a heart attack than the vegetarians. Vegetarians have more fiber in their diet. This, too, helps the arteries; as fiber passes through the digestive system, it absorbs fat and bile, and removes it from the body. In fact, the liver makes bile as one way of getting rid of cholesterol.

Both sugar and alcohol are converted to fat by the liver. Years of excessive alcohol or sugar consumption keep the liver producing excess fat and sending it out into the bloodstream for storage. Fasting or partial fasting is a well-tried method of ridding the body of extra fat, aiding the health of the circulation, and removing toxins. A general regimen for a healthy circulation is given in more detail in Chapter 7.

Positive components of the diet include leafy vegetables, fruits, nuts, and seeds. All food fiber is helpful, especially the soluble fiber found in fruits and vegetables. This fiber ties up the excess cholesterol that is dumped out of the liver as bile, and makes sure that it is passed out of the body through the intestines.

Besides reducing fat consumption to less than half the usual levels in the West, we should consider the types of fats we eat. Animal fats contribute to atherosclerosis, and it is now known that highly unsaturated vegetable oils such as soybean and safflower oils are not good for your circulation either, as they reduce the levels of the helpful HDL. The best oils are monounsaturated oils, especially olive oil.

We also know that whole grains are healthier than their refined counterparts; a cholesterol-lowering "drug" has been isolated from barley by scientists at the University of Wisconsin. Spices and herbs are, in general, flavorful and healthy additions to the diet, and some also lower cholesterol. It is, after all, among them that we find garlic.

Much research has focused on the fact that there are many individual nutrients in the diet that can help to protect the circulation, and that leave us vulnerable if they are missing in a refined and processed-food diet. These include the antioxidants—vitamins C and E, essential fatty acids, beta-carotene, zinc, copper, selenium, and magnesium. It is not easy, and certainly very expensive, to take all these "micronutrients" as supplements. But they can be found in natural, unrefined foods. The course is clear.

Garlic, as we shall see in the following chapters, has the most wide-ranging and beneficial effect on all of the processes described above. It significantly reduces the levels of cholesterol in the blood, especially the harmful, low-density lipoproteins, and it also increases the blood's tendency to dissolve clots. It seems tailor-made to help us in the dangerous position in which we now find ourselves, yet it is a natural and pleasurable part of our diet.

CHAPTER 5

Garlic, Heart Disease, and Cholesterol

Whether you take the advice of a cardiac specialist or a modern naturopath, you will be told that a fatty diet, smoking, eating animal products, and drinking large quantities of coffee are all hazardous practices for the circulation. However, if you travel to the south of France, or to Spain, you will find avid meat eaters, smokers everywhere, and not much guilt about coffee. By rights, the lovers of haute cuisine and the portly Italian and Spanish bourgeoisie should be at the top of the heart disease risk table. The fact is that they are towards the bottom. As you move from Northern to Southern Europe, there is a very clear decrease in the level of heart disease. The Greeks, and especially the Cretans, are level with the Japanese in having the least heart disease of all modern, developed nations.

GARLIC IS THE ANSWER

In looking for explanations to this phenomenon, scientists first thought that drinking wine, as opposed to beer or spirits, might be good for the heart, since those countries which drink more of it have lower levels of heart disease. This provoked a series of letters in the leading medical journal, *The Lancet,* during 1979. Some doctors who were familiar with the Mediterranean region wrote letters saying that since drinking wine and eating garlic go together there, it could be the latter which kept heart disease at bay. Following this, a thorough and careful analysis was made by statisticians at the University of Western Ontario in Canada. They confirmed that the more garlic a nation consumed, the lower its level of heart disease, and that there was a stronger association between garlic eating and cardiovascular health than wine drinking.

This is impressive. Nevertheless, the scientists admitted that there was similar epidemiological statistical evidence that it could also be the health-giving sun, the use of olive oil, the large amounts of fresh vegetables and salads, and probably the easy-going lifestyle or some other, unknown factor, which was responsible for the low rate of heart disease in Mediterranean countries.

What do the people of southern France or Spain have to say? What do they believe is their secret? If you ask them, they will tell you that the answer is garlic. After centuries of experience, they acknowledge garlic as the protector of their arteries. Indeed, many of them believe that its use in cooking was developed specifically to balance the diet and neutralize the harmful residues from the quantities of fats consumed. One can observe similar combinations of customs in other nations outside the Mediterranean area; the Koreans, for example, eat a lot of meat and take a great deal of garlic with it. Their heart disease level is also low. One rarely finds garlic on the tables of their neighbors, the Japanese, but they have a lighter diet, with fish instead of meat.

This kind of observation suggests, but by no means

proves, that garlic is effective in helping to reduce heart disease. To get more definite results, it would be necessary to take at least two groups of people who have similar lifestyles—except that one group eats garlic and the other does not—and then measure differences in their health and physical state. In the 1970s, Dr. G.S. Sainani and his colleagues at the Sassoon General Hospital in Pune, India, conducted a study of this type among the Jains, a unique religious community. All Jain families have similar vegetarian diets, except that some are accustomed to eating onions and garlic, while others adhere more strictly to their customs and traditionally abstain from them. Dr. Sainani assembled three groups of Jains who ate very similar amounts and types of food. However, in one group, each member had a weekly consumption of at least 600 g of onion and 50 g of garlic (this is the equivalent of around seventeen cloves, a fairly substantial quantity). The second group ate a weekly average of 200 g of onion and 10 g of garlic, while the third group ate none at all. It turned out that the amounts of cholesterol and fat in the Jains' blood matched their garlic and onion consumption very closely. The heavy garlic eaters had 25 percent less cholesterol than those who did not eat garlic. Since research has shown that a 10 percent drop in blood cholesterol reduces the risk of a heart attack by 20 percent, this is a major difference.

STUDIES PROVE GARLIC'S EFFECTIVENESS

As soon as scientists became aware that garlic might have a preventive action against heart disease, they began to test it in the laboratory. The first experiments were conducted at the Tagore Medical College, Rajasthan, India; at the University of Kerala, India; at Kyoto University, Japan; at the University of Wisconsin; and at Alcorn State University, Mississippi. These studies focused on the level of cholesterol in the blood. The Indian researchers already had a hunch that garlic could be protecting the circulation, because they found that in Indian traditional medicine, garlic is used to reduce fats in the blood. Indeed, it is stated in ancient texts that breastfeeding mothers should not eat a great deal of garlic because it might thin their milk.

The study of animals with heart disease has told us most of what we know about it, and confirmed many of the ideas for its treatment, including the use of garlic. Sadly, it is all too easy to give an animal atherosclerosis—one has only to feed it a typical modern diet, with plenty of butter and fatty meat. All the usual changes result—furring of the arteries, heart damage, and so on.

Garlic has been tested extensively on animals. The first observations were made in 1933 by scientists in Eastern Europe, who wanted to test the local belief that eating garlic stopped atherosclerosis in old age. They found that garlic could not only stop atherosclerosis in cats, but also reverse it. More precise modern studies over the last twenty years have shown that if rabbits, guinea pigs, and other animals are fed cholesterol or butter, together with their normal food, the cholesterol in their blood increases to abnormal levels. But if fresh garlic, garlic juice, garlic oil, or other garlic preparations are given as well, the increase is prevented completely. This has been demonstrated in nearly fifty published scientific studies.

For example, in a study at Alcorn State University, animals were fed their normal diet, together with cholesterol amounting to one percent of the total diet (an exceptionally high proportion). Some also received different kinds of dried garlic powder and extract. As expected, the cholesterol levels in the blood and the liver rose and stayed high. However, the various garlic powders and extracts reduced the cholesterol in the blood by about one-fourth, and in the liver by more than half, back to more or less normal levels.

Does this translate to an actual protection against heart disease? There have not been any studies comparing the number of heart attacks in animals fed garlic with the number of attacks in those who were not. However, several studies have examined the buildup of fats in the arteries. When a fatty diet is fed to animals, and their cholesterol rises as a result, this is reflected in more fats deposited inside the arteries. When garlic is added to the diet, it can stop the buildup of fatty blockages. A few studies have shown that the consumption of garlic can actually begin to reverse the fat buildup; that is, garlic can begin to clear fats out of the arteries, although this usually requires large amounts of garlic over a considerable period of time.

It was clear that fresh garlic powder and garlic oil were effective. There also were several similar studies involving pure allicin and diallyl disulfide—the main ingredient of garlic oil—which had similar results. These studies showed, therefore, that any odorous preparation of garlic would be effective against atherosclerosis. It made little difference whether the increase in fat in the body was produced by feeding the animals butter, lard, cholesterol, a great deal of sugar, or alcohol. All these unusual diets (unusual for the animals, that is!) produced raised levels of cholesterol and blood fat that could be reduced by feeding the animals garlic.

In another example, Professor Arun Bordia of the Rabindranath Tagore Medical College, Rajasthan, India, fed cholesterol-rich food to rabbits, and then gave them rather large quantities of garlic oil. He compared the results with those achieved by the drug clofibrate, one of the standard medical treatments given to people with high cholesterol. It turned out that the garlic was more effective than clofibrate in reducing the cholesterol that had accumulated in atherosclerotic plaques in the arteries, and also in reducing blood cholesterol levels.

This research also gives us the opportunity of understanding how garlic achieves this remarkable effect. According to scientists such as David Kritchevsky at the Wistar Institute in Philadelphia, garlic specifically slows down the manufacture of fats and cholesterol in the liver by slowing down the catalysts, and therefore the whole "production line" that makes the cholesterol. This means that cholesterol levels are reduced even when there is no surplus cholesterol in the diet, a fact that has been demonstrated in several studies on animals. For example, an investigation at the U.S. Department of Agriculture research laboratories in Madison, Wisconsin, involved feeding pigs their normal diet, together with garlic extract. The LDL, or "bad" cholesterol, fell by half, the helpful HDL cholesterol increased by 20 percent, and the production of these fats in the liver was also halved. It is interesting that the most powerful modern cholesterol-lowering drugs such as simvastatin or lovastatin also act on the body in a similar fashion.

It has been shown that animals fed with garlic excrete more bile as well as fat. Yet another mechanism may therefore be in operation, similar to the one used by the fibrate (fiber-like) category of milder modern drugs, such as gemfibrozil and clofibrate, used to reduce blood fats. Like them, garlic may help the liver to remove the extra cholesterol in the form of bile, and then eliminate the bile from the body.

Studies with animals also indicate that garlic therapy can actually remove fat from the walls of the blood vessels, and that about half the fatty plaques disappear. Two studies used the active ingredients of garlic in pure synthetic form. Scientists from China used pure allicin, and scientists from India used diallyl disulfide, on atherosclerotic animals. In both cases, they were able to prevent, and to some extent remove, fatty deposits from the arteries, including the arteries to the heart.

TESTING GARLIC ON HUMANS

Studies on animals are effective, but only studies on humans are really convincing. One factor to remember is that animal research always uses exaggeratedly high doses. Will garlic still work on people using normal daily amounts? The various clinical studies that have been carried out have addressed themselves to three main questions. Will garlic help individuals to dispose of extra fat after a fatty meal? Will it bring down the amounts of cholesterol and fats in people already suffering from excessive cholesterol and fat in their body, or from heart disease? Will it do so in those with normal levels?

Eating Garlic with a Fatty Meal

In India, where considerable scientific work on garlic has been performed, there have been studies on the effect of eating garlic and onions at the same time as fats. For example, in a study at the Cardiology Department of Rabindranath Tagore Medical College, a number of people were given a breakfast that included 100 g of butter. This led to a 10 percent rise in blood cholesterol a few hours afterwards, along with a drop of more than 20 percent in the fibrinolytic, or clot-removing, tendency of the blood. However, if garlic juice or garlic oil was also taken with the meal, these changes were completely prevented. In fact, the clot-removing tendency was increased by 20 percent. From this and other similar studies, we can conclude that eating garlic together with fatty food does help people to dispose of fats more easily, and to reduce their harmful after-effects.

This can make us feel better about adding garlic to our butter and serving garlic bread at meals. However, this should not be taken as license for an unrestrained fatty binge, relying on garlic as an antidote. The buildup of atherosclerosis is a deep, lifelong process, caused by daily heart-hurting habits continuing over many years. The changes are too great and irreversible for garlic alone to completely reverse. Garlic can help to stem the tide of fats coursing through the circulation, but it will not undo all the damage. For this, we need to address the root causes of atherosclerosis, and use garlic as an additional aid.

Effect of Garlic on High Cholesterol

When garlic is taken in a dose of at least one to two cloves a day (or the equivalent in product form), it will, according to some thirty clinical studies, reduce the amount of cholesterol in the blood by an average of 15 percent—enough to reduce the risk of a heart attack by 30 percent. A German study that was completed in 1988 looked at forty middle-aged people with high cholesterol levels. Their initial average was 7.6 mmol/l, or 295 mg/100 ml. Half of the group was given garlic products equivalent to one clove a day for three months. The other half was given a placebo—a neutral, look-alike preparation. The cholesterol levels of those taking garlic dropped steadily over the three-month period to an average of 6 mmol/l, or 233 mg/100 ml, a decrease of more than 20 percent. Those taking the placebo remained more or less the same. This is more than can be expected from regular, modern drugs. In addition, there were no reports of any kind of side effects, and those taking garlic also felt active and energetic by the end of the study.

The fact that there are so many studies of garlic is quite unusual in the world of plant medicine, which does not enjoy the massive financial support for research given to chemical drugs. Indeed, there are many official drugs on the market today that have not had the benefit of so many positive clinical studies. Moreover, the clinical studies today are of top quality. Here are two instructive examples. In 1990, a study was carried out by Professor F.H. Mader and colleagues, at many centers all over Germany, on 261 randomly selected patients with excess cholesterol. Some were given eight small garlic tablets (equivalent to less than a clove) per day, others a placebo. After sixteen weeks, the cholesterol levels of the garlic group were around 10 percent less, and the worse the problem was originally, the greater the reduction in cholesterol. Interestingly, very few of the participants in the trial noticed an odor from the tablets, though this is often a common complaint.

In a 1993 study by Dr. A.K. Jain and colleagues at Tulane University in New Orleans, subjects with moderately raised blood cholesterol were given an amount of garlic in tablet form similar to that used in Professor Mader's study. Like most of the previous studies, this one was double blind; that is, neither the researchers nor the participants knew who was receiving the garlic and who was receiving the placebo. Cholesterol fell by 6 percent, and LDL cholesterol by 11 percent. This is a small but worthwhile reduction, equivalent to that achieved by the milder of the modern cholesterol-lowering drugs. Again, hardly anyone noticed the odor because it was well-packaged inside coated tablets.

The Effect of Garlic on "Normal" Cholesterol

The question remains: Does garlic reduce cholesterol in everyone, whether they have raised levels or not, or does it only do so in those with problems? The answer is not so clear, since almost everyone in the modern world has levels which are higher than they should be, even those with so-called "normal" levels. However, it appears from the clinical studies that garlic does have some effect in all cases, but that the more cholesterol there is in the blood in the first place, the more it is reduced. For example, studies in India with people whose cholesterol levels were normal— below 5.2 mmol/l, or 200 mg/100 ml—found reductions of only a few percent, while studies of people in the risk area above 6.5 mmol/l, or 250 mg/100 ml, found a drop of up to one-fourth.

GARLIC AS A LONG-TERM REMEDY

Another conclusion to be drawn from the clinical research is that higher doses over longer periods produce better results. Garlic will start to work as soon as it is taken. However, the intake should continue for at least three months for more significant effects to occur. The evidence also shows that as soon as you stop taking garlic, the level of fat in the blood returns to what it was before. This fact is satisfying to scientists, since it demonstrates that it was the garlic which was effective, and not something else. To the rest of us, it says that garlic is not a magic potion which need only be taken now and again, but a medicinal food whose regular consumption should be an essential part of fat and cholesterol-lowering life habits.

This reinforcement was well demonstrated in a study by Professor E. Ernst of the University of Munich, published in the *British Medical Journal*. He chose patients who had high levels of cholesterol (above 6.7 mmol/l, or 260 mg/100 ml). Half were given a low-calorie diet for four weeks, and half were given the same diet together with a garlic preparation equivalent to just under a clove a day. Those on the diet had less cholesterol at the end of the period, but those taking garlic as well, even though the dose was modest, achieved a further 10 percent reduction. This study shows that garlic and a healthy diet should be used to help each other.

It is interesting to see which kind of cholesterol is affected. In the study by Professor Ernst, it was LDL, the unfriendly cholesterol, that was reduced; HDL remained unchanged. Professor Bordia, mentioned earlier, took sixty-two patients with heart disease and raised blood cholesterol, and examined the effect of giving them garlic oil and no other type of circulatory medicine. They were compared with a group of healthy people who also took garlic. Over eight months, the healthy people reduced their cholesterol by 15 percent; their LDL cholesterol was also reduced by 15 percent, and their HDL increased by nearly as much. In the group with heart disease, the cholesterol actually increased during the first month and then fell by 30 percent by the end of the period. The beneficial changes in LDL and HDL were correspondingly greater than in the normal group. Professor Bordia suggested that cholesterol may increase in heart patients for a short time after garlic is taken, since the garlic may be dislodging cholesterol from the artery walls. If this is true, it would imply that garlic is able to reverse atherosclerosis by removing fatty buildup. It would make garlic curative as well as preventive.

The medical dogma used to be that atherosclerosis was a one-way process that could be halted, but not reversed. Today, this is an open question. Diet and proper treatment can, it seems, reverse atherosclerosis to a greater or lesser extent, but it must be a serious effort involving a range of new life habits. Garlic has its place among them.

GARLIC AND THE GENERAL HEALTH
OF THE CIRCULATION

It is not easy to assess the health of the human circulatory system other than by measuring the various symptoms of degeneration that occur. The best-known symptom is, of course, the heart attack. However, it would require a long and expensive study to determine whether garlic reduces the number of heart attacks in a given group of people over many years. At a symposium on garlic in Germany in 1989, Professor Arun Bordia reported that he had carried out such a study over three years during the mid-1980s. The subjects were 430 patients who had already had one heart attack. They were all given standard medical treatment, but half were also given garlic oil. Over three years, there was, apparently, a drop of two-thirds in the incidence of a second heart attack in the group that had taken garlic.

It has been shown that garlic reduces a range of other symptoms of atherosclerosis. For a very long time, Russian doctors have been using garlic preparations as a standard treatment for atherosclerosis, especially in the elderly, and they have reported improvement of poor circulation in the legs and hands, fatigue, and so on. More recent studies on 300 patients in China, and on a similar number in India, found a rapid improvement in the symptoms of headache, chest pain, fatigue, loss of appetite, and digestive problems. However, when the garlic was withdrawn at the end of the study, the symptoms returned. Once more we see garlic's place as a long-term companion to health, rather than a short-term remedy.

One relatively common and distressing symptom of atherosclerosis is insufficient blood reaching the limbs. As this condition (known as *intermittent claudication*) becomes worse, it can prevent the sufferer from walking. Garlic has been found to be very helpful in such cases; it enhances the effect of exercise, diet, and other treatments, although it works best before the problem has become too severe. A study in Germany, published in the German journal *Medical Practice* in 1986, examined fifty-three patients before and after four weeks of treatment with doses of garlic equivalent to only a quarter of a clove per day. Tests were carried out on the flow of blood in the legs, and it was found to have improved by 50 percent. Nevertheless, a careful medical analysis of how the symptoms of atherosclerosis are affected by garlic is still needed.

GARLIC AND BLOOD PRESSURE

It is natural that if the blood vessels are narrowed by plaques and deposits, the heart will need to pump harder to keep the blood flowing through the body. Atherosclerosis can therefore lead to high blood pressure. This, in turn, puts an extra load on the heart and can further damage blood vessels, precipitate more atheromas (the plaques that build up in the vessels), and increase the risk of strokes. High blood pressure can also come from stress, tension, and a nervous disposition; from toxins in the body; from too much caffeine; or from waterlogging of the tissues, produced by too much salt in the diet or by hormonal imbalances. High blood pressure is a major cardiac risk factor, rivaling cholesterol. Normal blood pressure is 120 when the heart contracts (systolic), and 80 when it relaxes (diastolic), described as 120/80. A thirty-five-year-old man with blood pressure of 150/100 will, according to life insurance statistics, have a sixteen-year reduction in life expectancy. Can garlic help?

The answer is that it can, but its effect is mild. While garlic's action on blood fats and blood coagulation is as great as that of regular, modern drugs, this is not the case with blood pressure. Until recently, the only evidence available was in medical reports from Eastern Europe and Russia, where garlic is part of the regular treatment for high blood pressure. In the last few years, however, several well-conducted medical investigations have been completed in Europe. It was found that a drop of twelve to thirty millimeters in the systolic blood pressure and of seven to twenty millimeters in the diastolic could be obtained by the regular administration of garlic to patients with raised blood pressure. A smaller drop was likely in those with normal blood pressure.

For example, one study, completed in 1988, gave twenty patients tablets equivalent to about half a clove of garlic a day. They were compared with a similar group who received reserpine, a standard drug used to reduce high blood pressure. The study was a double-blind, meaning that neither the patients nor their doctors knew who was taking reserpine, and who was taking garlic. Within two weeks, the average systolic blood pressure in the garlic group dropped from 176 to 164, an average decrease of 7 percent; the diastolic came down from 99 to 85, a decrease of 14 percent. The effect of reserpine was more or less the same. Interestingly, only garlic reduced both blood pressure and blood fat. The conventional drugs used today to treat blood pressure are rather specific and do not affect cholesterol.

It is clear that fresh garlic, garlic oil, and other preparations are all effective. For example, a preparation of garlic oil tested on fourteen elderly women with high blood pressure brought the less severe cases down to normal. However, those whose conditions were due to kidney problems were not affected. In another study on eighty-two patients, pills of dried garlic were compared with placebos; blood pressure was reduced within the range already described, while the placebos had almost no effect. In both these studies, symptoms such as headache, dizziness, buzzing in the ears, and insomnia were considerably improved.

There is some uncertainty about how garlic acts on blood pressure. It used to be thought that it cleaned up putrefying bacteria in the intestine, the kind that change food constituents into various unwanted substances which raise blood pressure. Theories of intestinal hygiene were then at their peak. Today, such views have generally been superseded by the evidence that garlic affects the prostaglandins. These substances are present in the blood vessels and are in charge of opening, relaxing, or tightening them. If the vessels in the periphery of the body are relaxed, then there is less resistance to the blood flow. So far, there is quite a lot of evidence that garlic increases the flow of blood in these smaller vessels, and we also know that it affects the prostaglandin system. It is therefore reasonable to put the two together. There is also the traditional awareness that garlic makes a person sweat more and so dries out the body; this would also lower blood pressure.

This chapter has described many studies on groups of humans. However, the person taking his or her garlic is an individual. Just as the causes and results of circulatory disease differ in each case, so, too, will garlic's effects. There are indications that for some people it has a very dramatic therapeutic effect, while others do not seem to be greatly improved by it. The overall results, however, are overwhelmingly positive. You should use intelligence and discrimination in selecting any course of treatment and in assessing your personal reactions. In choosing garlic, you will run no risk of adverse effects. It is highly likely that your health will be improved, whether subtly or dramatically. So it is well worth the experiment.

CHAPTER 6

How Garlic Thins
The Blood

As we have said, blood clots in the arteries are like the pieces that stick to the inside of a kitchen waste pipe. They offer no danger when the blood still flows smoothly through open channels. However, as the vessels are narrowed, this life-saving mechanism operates against our interests. Major clots, or thromboses, can block the vital coronary arteries and cause a heart attack, or block one of the brain's blood vessels and cause a stroke, or block the vessels in the legs and cause venous thromboses and other problems. The clotting mechanism—especially the platelets—also plays a major part in the formation of the atherosclerotic plaques.

Garlic is one of the best anticlotting remedies that we know. There are several ways in which its effects can be calculated. The strength of the blood's clot-disintegrating mechanism can be measured. So, too, can the tendency of the platelets to clump together or, alternatively, the length of time taken by a sample of the blood to clot. The thinness of the blood, that is to say, its fluidity, can also be assessed; this is an important factor in high blood pressure, since the heart has to work harder to push heavier blood around the system.

BLOOD CLOTTING, DIETARY FAT, AND GARLIC

The amount and quality of your dietary fat intake has a powerful influence on the clotting tendency. Saturated fats and cholesterol increase blood clotting, while at the other end fish oils—and the EPA they contain—reduce it. Initial studies on the effects of garlic tried to find out whether it could remove the increased clotting created in the blood vessels by a fatty meal. Professor Arun Bordia, while initiating studies on cholesterol levels and garlic in animals, was at the same time the first to examine garlic's ability to return clotting to normal. He was impressed with the ancient Indian wisdom, dating back some two thousand years or more to Charaka, the father of traditional Indian medicine, that garlic helps to maintain the fluidity of the blood, strengthens the heart, and prolongs life. "But for its unpleasant odor," wrote Charaka, "garlic would be costlier than gold."

Professor Bordia fed small amounts of cholesterol to rabbits along with their normal diet for several months. Clots took twice as long as usual to dissipate during this period because of the increased cholesterol. However, if garlic oil was given along with the fatty diet, not only did the clot-removing activity *not* fall, but it actually increased by about 10 percent. In a similar study, Professor Bordia found that onion oil could achieve more or less identical effects. These observations have been repeated again and again in laboratories all over the world.

Other, similar studies were also carried out by Professor Bordia and other researchers on humans. Again, clot-dissolving activity began to fall after a fatty meal. This could be observed easily and immediately, so it was a relatively simple matter to assess whether garlic could block this effect. Once more it was found that both garlic and onion not only stopped the fall but even increased clot-dissolving activity. For example, a group of studies was carried out in 1969 by Professor I.S. Menon, then a research fellow at the Royal Victoria Infirmary in Newcastle upon Tyne. They were published in the prestigious *British Medical Journal.* Professor Menon's inspiration came, he said, from "a casual remark by a patient that in France, when a horse develops clots in the legs, it is treated by a diet of garlic and onions." In this study, twenty-two patients who were convalescing in his hospital were given a fatty breakfast. After two hours, samples of their blood were taken and the clot-dissolving activity was found to be 25 percent lower than before eating the meal. However, if the patients were then given two ounces of fried or boiled onion with the same meal, the activity increased by 50 percent.

In a similar study carried out by Dr. R.C. Jain in India, ten healthy people were given a very buttery breakfast and their blood coagulation time was checked. Three hours later this time was checked again, and, as expected, the clot-dissolving activity was down from about eighty-four units to forty-three. However, if they took the same breakfast, this time with garlic added to the butter, clot-dissolving activity went up to eighty-six units. Their blood would normally clot in an average of 4 minutes and 15 seconds. After the breakfast it took only 3 minutes, 41 seconds. However, if garlic was added to the butter it took 5 minutes, 7 seconds to clot, slower than normal.

Garlic's effect on blood clotting is indeed dramatic. Its action takes place within a few hours, it is easy to measure, and it is major. Unlike cholesterol levels, which are quite hard to change unless treated over long periods of time, ingestion of garlic leads to large and immediate reductions in the clotting tendency. This is partly due to the effectiveness of garlic and partly due to the fact that clotting generally responds more easily to changes in diet and other factors; a good bout of exercise will also produce an obvious reduction, and modern anticholesterol drugs such as the fibrates will also reduce clotting tendency along with the cholesterol levels.

Clinical research has demonstrated that garlic increases fibrinolytic (clot-dispersing) activity and clotting times in those suffering from heart disease or atherosclerosis, as well as in healthy people. For example, a study published in 1981 in the journal *Atherosclerosis* involved twenty subjects who all had coronary heart disease, and had all had previous heart attacks. Their clot-dissolving activity started in the morning at sixty-two units and rose slightly during the day to seventy units. However, if they were given either fried or raw garlic, the activity increased within six hours to over 100 units. When they were given garlic for one month continuously, it went up even higher, to 122 units with fresh garlic and 110 with fried. The garlic was stopped at that point, and within two weeks the clot-dissolving activity was back to the original level.

An analysis of fifteen similar clinical studies involving hundreds of subjects shows garlic increasing the clot-dispersing ability of the blood by an average of 60 percent. This could be achieved after taking garlic for only one day, although the effects also tended to increase with time. When the garlic was removed from the diet, clot-dispersing activity gradually fell back to what it was before. In this case, fresh and fried garlic were found to work more or less equally well. Other reports confirm that garlic oil, garlic extract, fresh or dried garlic, and onion or onion oil were all similarly effective at thinning the blood.

All these observations were so remarkable and well defined that in 1981, *The Lancet* announced in an enthusiastic editorial that it had high hopes for a natural reduction in blood clotting by dietary factors such as garlic. As is clear from the research described above, onion can also affect the clotting process, perhaps almost as strongly as garlic. However, onion cannot replace garlic as a treatment for the heart, as it does not have its other effects, such as lowering the levels of fats and cholesterol; it is not such a good, all-around remedy.

GARLIC, PLATELETS, AND THE STICKINESS OF THE BLOOD

Platelets are the small cell fragments that are the advance guard of the clotting process. They are acutely sensitive to disturbances and chemical triggers that might indicate a wound or break. If such a trigger occurs, they immediately clump together, releasing a cascade of trigger substances that initiate the clotting process locally. A variety of influences are known to make them clump together; these include the presence in the blood of protein fibers called *collagen*, which are normally part of the connective tissues and should not intrude into in the blood vessels unless there is some kind of fracture. That well-known biological alarm bell, adrenaline, also causes the platelets to clump, a mechanism obviously intended to prepare the body for possible injury.

The speed at which the platelets clump together is a very sensitive indicator of how sticky the blood is, how soon it will clot, and the likelihood of the clotting occurring where it is not wanted—that is, in the atherosclerotic blood vessels. Atherosclerosis is always accompanied by some increase in blood stickiness. The speed of clumping is also the easiest, most reliable, and quickest of all tests of the effectiveness of garlic. One only has to give a person garlic to eat, wait a short while, and take a blood sample. Then it is a simple matter to check under a microscope how fast the platelets clump when triggered to do so by, for example, adrenaline.

Such tests have been carried out by many scientists. These include Dr. David Boullin, who was working as a member of a Medical Research Council hematology team at Oxford in 1981. He found that the prevention of clumping is noticeable within an hour after garlic is eaten, and that it continues for three to four hours, after which the clumping returns to normal. This gives us a clear picture of the rate at which garlic enters the body, acts therapeutically, and is then removed in the same way as other foods or medicines.

What is even more interesting is that the doses of garlic needed to significantly reduce platelet clumping are low. The reduced stickiness of platelets can be noticed in the blood of someone who has eaten less than half a clove of garlic. Since this restricts blood clotting for a few hours, then one clove per day, or its equivalent, divided into morning and evening doses, would be the safe minimum necessary to generate noticeable results. Indeed, patients with high blood cholesterol have been given tablets equivalent to only one quarter of a clove of garlic per day for three months and their stickiness and clumping tendency measured. Gradually, over the three-month period, the clumping tendency was reduced by 20 percent and the stickiness by around 30 percent. Again, studies have shown that fresh garlic, extracts, and garlic oil are all effective.

Because this method is such a simple and sensitive barometer of garlic's effects on the body, it has attracted a considerable world research effort. The goal has been to identify which compounds within garlic affect the platelet system, and to determine how they achieve this. In each case, scientists have broken down and refined garlic into its component parts and have tested each for blood-clotting effects. Finally, they have arrived at the single pure compound that they consider the most effective. Unfortunately, though many research teams have expended a great deal of effort, they have all arrived at different conclusions. The results are summarized in Table 6.1. At present, we do not know which of these compounds is the most effective. It is only safe to say that each is highly

TABLE 6.1. GARLIC COMPOUNDS THAT AFFECT BLOOD CLOTTING

Research Team	Compounds Discovered	Comment
Dept of Biochemistry, George Washington University School of Medicine, Washington, D.C.	Adenosine Allicin Dimethyl trisulphide (and related poly-sulphides)	Present in fresh garlic juice, extract, etc.
Dept of Pathology, College of Medicine, University of Utah	Allicin	As above
Institute of Pharmaceutical Biology, University of Munich	Ajoene Vinyl 1–2, dithiin Diallyl disulphide	Not in fresh garlic. May be in fried garlic
Dept of Physiology, Nikon University School of Medicine, Tokyo	Methyl allyl trisulphide (MATS)	Present at around 5% in garlic oil
Dept of Chemistry, University of Delaware	Diallyl trisulphide Vinyl 1–2, dithiin 1,5, hexadienyl-trisulphide	Not in fresh garlic. May be in fried garlic
Dept of Chemistry, State University of New York, Albany	Ajoene	As above
University of Cologne	Adenosine	As above

active. How much there is of each compound in the different kinds of garlic or garlic products is also hard to say. It is interesting to note that at least two of these compounds, ajoene and methyl allyl trisulfide (MATS) are now undergoing tests as possible pure and safe pharmaceuticals against blood clotting.

A great deal of knowledge has now accumulated concerning how garlic and its constituents work to prevent blood clotting. It is generally agreed the sulfur compounds interfere with the chemical machinery that makes the prostaglandins, which control the way platelets clump. It is interesting that low-dose aspirin, the remedy most often given by doctors as a long-term preventive against excessive clotting, works in a similar manner. Comparative trials of aspirin and garlic show that, at recommended doses, garlic has at least as much effect on blood clotting as aspirin.

Garlic influences the prostaglandins in the walls of the blood vessels as well as in the platelets themselves. It increases the production of prostacyclin, which limits clotting, and reduces that of thromboxane A_2, which encourages it. There may be some concern that blood clotting is an essential process that should not be interfered with. However, this is unfounded, since the clotting tendency of people in modern, developed countries is already too high, probably because of the diet and the fatty deposits in the blood vessels. Garlic simply lowers clotting tendency to a more normal level. There is no evidence that people who eat a very large amount of garlic in their daily diet have a problem with too much bleeding. In various studies, people have been given the equivalent of two heads of garlic a day (about twenty cloves) for months, without showing any tendency to bleed excessively. However, it would be well to note that if garlic is being taken along with aspirin and anticoagulant drugs, the effects can reinforce each other. This will not normally be harmful, but should perhaps be avoided in special situations such as surgery.

We can now understand the observations made by the herbalists of the past that garlic thins the blood. It has been amply confirmed by numerous scientific studies. Even more than that, some of the anticlotting compounds in garlic are so active that they are now being investigated for possible development as new anticlotting drugs. This should give us even more apprieciation for the surprising medical power of this remarkable plant.

CHAPTER 7

Garlic, a Healthy Diet,
and Your Heart

In this chapter, we are going to look beyond garlic, and touch briefly on some of the other principles of self-care that we will need to utilize to keep the heart pumping and the circulation moving freely without problems. These principles go well with garlic and come from the same natural medicine tradition. This tradition states that we can rely on nature to provide us with answers to our health problems, but we must learn nature's messages. Human culture always utilized a huge knowledge of the health properties of various foods and diets; the medicinal properties of hundreds of common herbs, spices, and medicinal foods; the ways to treat common health problems within the household; how to build resistance; how people differ; and how each kind of person should live in order to maximize health and life span. Unfortunately, our modern civilization has lost much of this knowledge and at the same time created health problems, such as by processing foods and adding pesticides and other toxic substances to them. In this chapter, we will briefly introduce some of this basic folk knowledge, in particular that of the right foods to eat to protect the heart. As we shall see, we do not need to feel that we must return to primitive times. Science is gradually coming round to agreeing that natural, wholesome foods are best for us.

GARLIC AS A PART OF PREVENTIVE HEART CARE

Garlic is certainly useful, but it cannot purge the world of its major health problems unaided. It is not a panacea. Those who really know how to use it regard garlic as an important dietary tool, which should take its place in the self-care tool kit along with all the other aids that nature has been thoughtful enough to provide. Garlic cannot be expected to provide the whole answer after the damage has been done. In fact, this would be treating it just like a modern drug, and it is such drug-dependent attitudes which have, to some extent, created the problems of heart disease in the first place. Such attitudes hold that it does not really matter what you do or how you live, because there will always be a pill available to put you right. It is now becoming clearer every day that only self-care can really halt the degenerative process within the circulation.

It is unlikely that garlic alone will lower the level of heart disease to that of vegetarians or the Japanese who follow a traditional diet, but its use as part of an overall self-care regimen should be able to achieve this. Moreover, it is not only the health of the arteries that will be improved. Just as garlic itself has a range of benefits, so too will the principles of health care that we are about to outline. Common problems such as fatigue, headaches, obesity, colitis, arthritis, *Candida*, hypoglycemia, cancer, and low-ered immunity can all be prevented, and often actually cured, in this way.

Some may react against the idea of garlic as a medicine.

This is largely a cultural problem. The traditional, well-tried methods of maintaining health, which are part of our national heritages, have been largely lost. Gone too, at least in Northern Europe and America, is the automatic use of garlic and other medicinal foods. To reestablish their use in your personal life may require a little more effort and special interest. But the principles of self-care are coming back. Even government agencies encourage it more than they did ten years ago. Eventually, garlic and other medicinal foods will make a full return to popularity.

TOWARDS A PROGRAM FOR PREVENTION

The first way to protect the circulation is simply to stop abusing it. Modern life presents us with a constant succession of influences that weigh on our vascular systems. Indeed, we regard high blood pressure and heart attacks as more or less inevitable for adult males, much like tuberculosis in the last century or malaria in the tropics. Yet the Japanese do not suffer from atherosclerosis unless they emigrate to a Western country. They eat less than one-third of the fat that Westerners eat, and the traditional Japanese diet has no dairy products, meat products, sugar, bread, or cakes.

The blood pressure of the Solomon Islanders, the Australian aborigines, and other such groups goes down with age, not up. They eat no salt. The Eskimos eat a great deal of fat, but live without heart problems; however, they are protected by fish oil, and they, too, eat no salt or dairy products. From very extensive reviews of who is, and who is not, vulnerable to heart disease, we learn of the role of smoking; the dangers of stress, anxiety, and tension; the essential need for exercise; the need for vitamins, essential fatty acids, fiber, and other food factors; and the subsidiary risks of coffee, pesticides, and the like. The importance of all of these factors has been confirmed by extensive work in the laboratory.

It is interesting that this entire research effort is steadily drawing us towards conclusions reached long ago by Hippocrates, Galen, the ancient Egyptian physicians, and the preventive advice given by naturopathy, herbalism, and traditional Chinese and Indian medicine. They have always emphasized the necessity for moderation, a wholesome diet, exercise, and an easy-going approach to life. (See *The Need For Exercise* inset on page 69.) Here are the main items to consider in relation to cardiovascular health. You will know which are most relevant to you.

SUGGESTIONS FOR A HEALTHY DIET

Doctors are now unanimous in recommending a reduction in saturated fats. Various conservative pronouncements by the health authorities, such as the U.S. National Cholesterol Education Program's "Step I" diet, advise a drop in fatty meats and full-fat dairy products to reduce fat intake from the usual American high level of 37 percent of the diet to 30 percent. Saturated fats should be reduced from 15 percent to 10 percent. They also recommend a modest increase in consumption of fruits, vegetables, and fiber-containing foods. This is a start, but it is certainly not enough to make a serious impact on your clogged arteries. If followed, this diet will achieve a mere 10 to 20 percent drop in heart disease. A proper consideration of the risks must tell us that in order to achieve a substantial reduction, it is absolutely necessary to create new eating habits. If, to take the extreme case, the whole population were to turn vegetarian, cholesterol levels would be reduced by 25 percent, the blood-clotting tendency would fall considerably, blood pressure would come down to normal, and deaths from heart attacks would be halved.

THE NEED FOR EXERCISE

Proper exercise is one of the most important keys to a healthy heart. It is advisable to exercise vigorously at least once a day. (Traditionally, exercise is described as vigorous if it makes you sweat.) The amount of exercise you should get depends on how fit you are. If you are not fit, you should build up to it very gradually.

Exercise is more beneficial if it is regular and rhythmic. Swimming, jogging, dancing, skiing, digging, cycling, yoga, and tai chi are all excellent forms of exercise. The body does better on less intense exercise for a longer time than on very intense exercise for a short period, followed by inactivity. Likewise, exercise should be kept up as far as possible throughout life. There are many stories of keen athletes whose first heart attack happened after they gave up all sports and went to fat in their middle age. It would have been better to have done less, but to have kept it going more regularly.

The benefits of exercise are well known. Cholesterol levels are substantially decreased. The clot-removing activity of the blood is increased and clots are less likely to form because the blood is thinner and flows faster. Arteries expand, offering less resistance; blood pressure falls; stress is dissipated; the heart becomes slower and stronger; and there is some evidence of a reversal of atherosclerotic plaques in the arteries. The list could continue. Numerous studies have concluded that regular exercise reduces the risk of a heart attack by at least half.

Conventional physicians know very little about the more radical natural approaches. Indeed, most physicians cannot handle the more therapeutic "Step II" diet recommended by the National Cholesterol Education Program for the treatment of people suffering from high levels of cholesterol, which requires a reduction of saturated fat to only 7 percent of the diet, and will just prescribe drugs or call in a dietitian. For more serious dietary changes, you will need to work out completely different eating habits from the standard American diet.

It may not be necessary to become a vegetarian, but it is necessary to return to a more natural, whole food diet— one that includes garlic. Here are some guidelines for a diet that really will make a difference.

Carbohydrates

Carbohydrates include all the sweet or starchy, energy-giving food substances in potatoes, bread, pasta, rice, and other grains, and in sugar-containing foods. They are the mainstay of your diet and they should make up two-thirds of everything you eat. From the heart's point of view, all carbohydrates are perfectly satisfactory, provided they are not refined or "empty." Natural unrefined and unprocessed carbohydrates have 10 percent of their weight as fiber, vitamins, essential minerals, and fats, all of which are needed for proper health and metabolism. So carbohydrates should be based on whole grains or vegetables in which the entire package of food components is present.

It is advisable to be modest with carbohydrate consumption, as excess will be converted to fat in the body. However, there is less concern with excess carbohydrates than with excess fats. In addition, you can eat "whole food" carbohydrates more freely than refined carbohydrates, which are more easily converted to fats. Here are some suggestions for carbohydrate consumption:

- Avoid white flour in bread, cakes, crackers, and so forth. It deprives you of valuable fiber and vitamins. As it is too easily transformed into sugars in the digestive system, it puts a strain on the pancreas, which has to dispose of the sudden excess. It is also more readily converted into fat.

- Avoid sweets, chocolates, cakes, custard, puddings, and so forth. These also add "empty" carbohydrates which lead to higher amounts of fat in the blood.

- Use bread, pasta, and other foods made with whole wheat flour. Whole wheat, oats, barley, corn, buckwheat, rye, millet, brown rice, tapioca, and semolina are unrefined sources of carbohydrates that can be the basis of many dishes, either as whole grains, flakes, or flours. Oats and barley contain fiber and other special ingredients that lower cholesterol in the body. A breakfast of oatmeal is a vast improvement on eggs and bacon.

- Lentils, peas, beans, and nuts contain a great deal of beneficial carbohydrates.

- If you have a sweet tooth, eat dried fruit, molasses, or a little honey or brown sugar. Carob chocolate is almost indistinguishable from ordinary chocolate, but without the heavy saturated fats.

- Garlic goes well in pickles, sauces, and dips for use with whole meal bread. A classic Middle Eastern dip, which is excellent for the circulation, consists of olive oil, squeezed lemon, garlic, and marjoram, mixed together. In the Mediterranean, garlic is used liberally on country bread, and in pasta sauces, risottos, and rice dishes.

Protein

Protein provides the essential "building blocks" for the body. However, it should take second place to carbohydrates in the diet. The average Western adult eats too much protein, which can lead to overweight and excess animal fat. It can create too much waste in the blood, loading the body with toxins, and sometimes encouraging diseases such as allergies, arthritis, and digestive problems. You can gradually adjust to eating less protein, to your benefit. Here are some suggestions:

- Eat much less meat. Try to avoid fatty meat, hamburgers, hot dogs, sausages, pork, and bacon altogether. Don't eat meat pies, chicken pies, or processed forms of meat products. These may contain poor quality meat, plus a lot of unwanted fats, salt, and other additives.

- If you eat meat, make sure that it is as lean as possible, or try meat substitutes. Better still, leave meat out of your diet altogether, and move towards obtaining your proteins from natural seeds and grains, or from fish.

- Use vegetarian pies or spreads instead of meat.

- Reduce the amount of eggs you eat. One a day is too many, especially if they come from conventional farms. Try to buy free-range eggs if you can; they are better for your health, since they contain more nutrients and less agricultural chemicals and antibiotics—they taste better, too.

- Avoid full-fat cheeses, such as Cheddar, Stilton, and cream cheese. Try to eat less cheese and, if necessary, use cottage cheese or feta cheese. Use light cheese products and reduced-fat soft cheeses. Try kefir and live natural yogurt.

- Avoid cow's milk; adults don't need it. Try tofu and soy milk instead.

- Eat more fish, especially mackerel, herring, tuna, sardines, and salmon, which are all rich in fish oil.

- Nuts are rich in protein and make very good spreads.

- Try to eat a continuously changing variety of legumes and seeds; they are the mainstay of vegetarian protein sources. These include split peas, lentils, lima beans, broad beans, chickpeas, hummus, tahini, soybeans, sunflower seeds, mung beans, and the "macrobiotic meat," adzuki beans. Sesame seeds have more protein per unit of weight than meat.

- Garlic goes well with lean meat, especially in French garlic sauces; it also goes well with fish, especially when combined with parsley. You can add crushed garlic and dill to cottage cheese to give it a rich, aromatic flavor. Crushed garlic is a necessary addition to hummus (chickpea paste), tahini (Greek and Middle Eastern ground sesame seeds), and cooked soybeans. Add a little garlic to nut roasts, casseroles, and lentil pies.

Fats

Fats are the major problem for the circulation. Try to reduce fat to no more than 15 percent of your diet. This means rarely frying food—*never* deep-frying—and drastically reducing the fatty sources of protein, particularly dairy products and meat. Saturated fats, particularly from animal sources, are regarded as the worst foods for the heart. Here are some suggestions for reducing fats in your diet:

- Avoid saturated fats as much as possible. Reduce consumption of animal products, especially cream and other rich dairy products. Always use oil—never butter—for cooking and frying, and try not to heat oil to too high a temperature, because unsavory and unhealthy burnt components can be created.

- For all-around kitchen use, the best oil is olive oil, because it is monounsaturated and less refined than other oils. You can cook with it, but it should not be heated to too high a temperature. Apart from olive oil, sesame oil is excellent, and can be heated. Otherwise use soybean, sunflower, corn, and safflower oils. For salads, dips, and so forth, always use virgin olive oil. Try to use cold-pressed, first pressed, or virgin vegetable oils. This means that they are pressed in the traditional way, without refining. Refining drastically reduces the quantity of beneficial and necessary oils, and converts them into unnecessary oils. It also destroys natural antioxidants in the oils. Cold-pressed oils are not widely available, so look for them in health food stores.

- Avoid spreading butter or heavy fat spreads on bread. Use olive oil-based margarine if possible. This should be available in health food stores. Use vegetable oil instead of margarine wherever possible in pastry. Consider other spreads such as tofu, tahini, nut butters, and vegetable spreads as alternatives to margarine.

- Avoid hidden fats in processed products. For example, potato chips, snacks, and cookies can have a great deal of fat in them, often of very poor quality. Don't eat these products.

- Don't forget that all vegetables and grains have a little oil in them, and seeds more, enough for your requirements. It is not necessary to add oil to your diet if you already have a balanced and varied diet with plenty of vegetables, seeds, and grains, especially if you are treating a heart problem.

- Garlic is fried in oil, often with onion, in Indian and Chinese cooking and in other ethnic dishes. The oil is then used as the basis for numerous dishes such as curries. Virgin olive oil, together with lemon, cider vinegar, garlic, and a little mustard and herbs, is the best basic salad dressing. Add fresh garlic to a little olive oil and spread on fresh whole-meal bread before warming it in the oven. This is not very different from garlic butter. Garlic goes well with lemon or soy sauce on avocados, which are rich in natural oil.

Fiber, Vitamins, and Minerals

Fiber refers to all the indigestible material contained in vegetable sources of food. It provides the bulk, or "roughage," that the digestive system requires to work properly. Lack of fiber in the diet is a modern phenomenon, since refining and processing removes it from food. Soluble fiber, found in oats, fruits, and vegetables, is especially important to those at risk from heart disease because it binds fats and cholesterol and removes them from the body. (The modern fibrate-type, cholesterol-lowering drugs are, incidentally, derived from food fiber and work in this manner.) Fruits and vegetables should be the mainstay of a diet for a healthy circulation. Besides the fiber, fruits and vegetables contain most of the essential micronutrients, such as antioxidants, vitamins, and minerals, that protect our health.

Here are some tips for adding fiber, vitamins, and minerals to your diet:

- There should be around 40 g of fiber in the diet per day. Leafy vegetables contain 5 to 9 g of fiber in every 100 g, whole wheat flour 9 g. Vegetables and salads should be regarded as an essential part of the diet, not as decorative accessories. Ideally, for treating circulatory problems, all meals should be based on vegetables, served either as salads or lightly cooked. The minimum should be one vegetable-based meal every day.

- Vegetables should be as fresh as possible. A sodden mass of canned or overcooked vegetables will not give you much in the way of nutrients. Vegetables like spinach should be cooked very lightly, by boiling, steaming, or braising for the minimum time. The best vegetables are organically grown, fresh vegetables in salad. If you can't find them, at least buy the freshest vegetables you can. However, don't undo all the good of your salads with lashings of mayonnaise or heavy dressings.

- It is unnecessary and expensive to take tablets made of fiber or to pour bran on your foods. If your daily diet contains a sufficient intake of vegetables, salads, whole grains, and fruits, it will not be necessary to add extra fiber. The nutritional value of poor quality, empty, refined foods cannot be fully restored by adding fiber and vitamins. Many other nutrients will still be missing.

- Vegetables that are particularly good for the circulation include all those that are "heating"—that is, that make you sweat a little, warm the body, and open the blood vessels. These include radishes, onions, hot peppers, and, of course, garlic. Garlic is a rich source of minerals and also contains trace elements such as germanium and selenium.

Salt

Since salt raises blood pressure, it is one of the major risk factors in heart disease. It has now been demonstrated conclusively that it is unnecessary on health grounds to add any salt to the diet. It used to be thought that the body needs salt to make up its losses from sweating. However, scientists have now found that the body actually needs very little salt, and there is enough in the diet already without adding more. Sweating only removes excess salt. In hot countries, those people who don't eat salt sweat pure water; those who do eat salt, sweat salt.

You would be well advised to reduce salt in your diet. Fortunately, there is a range of salt substitutes available, including and especially potassium salt, which does not increase blood pressure. Spices and herbs can be a healthy and flavorful salt substitute.

Garlic provides a rich rather than a salty flavor. Mixing it with other herbs such as parsley and basil produces such an interesting aroma that the addition of salt becomes less relevant.

Drinks

Coffee is not particularly helpful to the heart, and if possible you should reduce the amount you drink. Two and a half cups of coffee will double the level of adrenaline circulating in the blood. It also makes the heart itself more sensitive to the damage caused by the adrenaline excess. In others words, coffee and stress together are an unwholesome combination. (See *Relaxation and Letting Go* inset on page 78.) Decaffeinated coffee or coffee made from grains, dandelion, or chicory can be convenient substitutes.

Tea is also caffeinated, though it has tannins which are known to help remove fats in the digestive system. Black

RELAXATION AND LETTING GO

Stress can damage the circulation, whether dietary or other factors are working for or against it. In fact, the discovery of the effects of stress arose through a study which tried to determine why some people with a great deal of furring of the arteries succumbed to heart trouble while others with similar arteries were free of it. The answer lay in the different ways in which the people reacted to the challenges of life. Those people, especially men, who are irritable, anxious, constantly over-stimulated, under strain, perfectionist, tense, clock-watching, ambitious, impatient, or angry all suffer from too much physiological arousal. Their adrenaline is constantly circulating and their stress hormones are erratic; the result is narrowed arteries, higher blood pressure, heart damage, and twice the risk of heart disease. The risk of other diseases is also increased, since stress reduces the body's immunity. Surveys have found that two out of three visits to general practitioners in modern cities are made for stress-related conditions. The natural systems that make us alert when faced with danger have themselves become dangerous by responding so relentlessly to the challenges and disturbances of modern life. There are several answers to this problem.

Cardiologists like Professor Peter Nixon at Charing Cross Hospital in London now teach relaxation and counseling to cardiac patients as a frontline defense against internal alarm systems. It has been found that if the adrenaline can sometimes be switched off completely, it is able to function in a less damaging manner. Dr. Chandra Patel and other researchers at St. George's Hospital Medical School in London were the first to demonstrate, more than twenty years ago, that regular deep relaxation sessions will reduce blood pressure by 15 to 20 percent, and cholesterol levels by at least 10 percent. In 1990, Dr. Dean Ornish published a paper in *The Lancet* demonstrating that lifestyle changes that feature techniques of deep relaxation, counseling, dietary changes, and exercise can actually reverse the buildup of atherosclerosis in the arteries.

Relaxation training is easily undertaken. It is taught in many health centers and in private groups, and can even be learned from audio or video tapes. The states produced are the beginning stages of meditation, akin to the deep peace one feels when absorbed in pleasant daydreams or a beautiful piece of music. Once you learn how to relax deeply, the memory of the state will be with you as a permanent assistance in stressful moments. Sometimes relaxation training can be helped by biofeedback. This involves using a small monitor, by which you can check on your level of relaxation and guide yourself deeper.

Counseling is also very useful. Heart attack patients are often brought together in guided groups in order to discuss their problems. The support offered by such groups is known to help prevent recurrences. Counseling ranges from the provision of a good listener to whom one can unburden oneself, all the way to psychotherapy. It has become common practice for large corporations to have a free counseling service available to executives so as to reduce the buildup of stress.

A more profound method of mental control is meditation, of which there are many different techniques. Here the relaxation is deepened so as to enter states of quiet watchfulness. One modern version, called autogenic training, employs the use of affirmative statements about the health of the body and the circulation. These act much like hypnosis in releasing interior tensions and improving bodily states. There is considerable evidence of the positive physiological effects of meditation on the circulation and the blood. Moreover, these methods are very helpful in giving you more control over your lifestyle and habits.

There is a deeper dimension to stress which is only now beginning to be appreciated. It is that sense of being out of touch with yourself. It is a lack of love in your life, from you to others, others to you, and you to yourself. The therapy is connectedness with life and emotional balance. This is not something which is easily learned through techniques, or easily won even in counseling, although they do help. Nor can the solution be prescribed—it is an individual process. However, it is important to remember that to give enough space to relationships to others and to oneself, and to let go and take life as it comes, may be as important to the heart as any technique or diet.

tea has been found to reduce cholesterol in the body. Green tea, as drunk in the Far East, is even better as a cholesterol-reducing drink. Although you can buy special slimming teas containing Chinese green tea, you can save the money—ordinary green tea is just as good. The current enthusiasm for herb teas greatly increases the range of hot drinks available. Three widely available, tasty herbal teas can help to lower blood pressure. They are lime flower, hibiscus flower, and mint teas.

Alcohol is chemically from the same family as fat, so the same rules apply to both. However, a little red wine is said to be beneficial to the heart.

SOME SUGGESTIONS FOR CHANGING YOUR DIET

The major difficulty in improving your diet is trying to break old habits. Unfortunately, many people only summon the will to change after some obvious symptom of heart disease occurs—such as a heart attack—and the driving force is then fear. It is much better to act before trouble develops. Nevertheless, it is never too late to make an improvement. The change can be made in various ways. A period in a health resort, a visit to a naturopath, or a supervised period of fasting and a complete clean-up, can be an excellent way to start. It will make you feel good; a multitude of small symptoms disappear and general vitality is restored, and this provides the motivation to continue.

Another way is to change your diet gradually, by substitution. Keep the same dietary patterns but change the items you eat: substitute brown bread for white, oil for butter, fish for meat, rice for french fries, and so on. You can move imperceptibly towards a whole food diet without noticing it.

A key aspect of revising your diet is to be in touch with your food; regard it as important, interesting, and a source of pleasure. Be aware of what you eat and explore new foods with a sense of experiment and adventure. Cooking is also a very relaxing process. It benefits your heart when you relax and spend some time in simple food preparation, and it benefits even it more when you eat your own healthy creations. Make your food pleasant to look at and taste, and involve friends and family in the proceedings. One interesting way of doing this is to cook foreign foods; Chinese, Indian, Japanese, Greek, or Mexican foods often contain the healthy ingredients we have been discussing.

One common pitfall is to pay too much attention to advertisements. The end result is the substitution of one set of packaged, instant, processed foods for another. It is a common reflex in our modern world to respond to all changes required of us by buying something. In the case of food, it is helpful to become less of a purchaser and more of a preparer. This shifts the emphasis away from processed foods towards real foods—grains, vegetables, legumes, fresh fish, and so forth. Try the experiment of not buying any factory-prepared and processed foods at all. It will benefit your health, your budget, and your entire way of life. A rich world of direct contact and experience with what is, after all, the basis of your life, may be revealed. I personally enjoy baking bread, which I do every couple of days, using home-grown organic wheat. Early in the morning, rhythmically kneading the dough, feeling its soft and changing textures, smelling its rich odors, experimenting with combinations of different seeds, grains, and herbs, listening to the chorus of birds outside, and the quiet in the house: this is one of the high points of my day. The next one, of course, is eating the result for breakfast.

Finally, there is perhaps the most important consideration of all in changing dietary habits—children. Heart attacks at age 40 have their origins in the eating habits established in childhood. Children will generally like the food common to the society around them; responding to the world's persuasion, they will be drawn to a diet of sweet, packaged, and processed foods. At home, however, they should receive only real, nutritious foods. Parents who say, "I've tried them with vegetables, they won't eat them," reveal resignation and their own basic lack of interest. Try getting your children to share in the adventure of discovering real food. If you are consistent and imaginative about this, they will like and ask for whole food, and regard junk foods as suspect.

SPECIAL FOODS THAT HELP THE HEART

All the alliums besides garlic are helpful. Onions, for example, have similar, though weaker, effects on the circulation. Chives and leeks should not be ignored. Of the other vegetables, radishes, cauliflower, and Brussels sprouts are useful in detoxifying the liver.

The minerals magnesium, potassium, and manganese are of special importance to the heart and circulation. These can be found in seeds such as sesame and sunflower, molasses, dark green leafy vegetables like spinach and parsley, and apple juice or cider vinegar.

Spices and herbs can be very helpful. For example, ginger stimulates and calms the digestion, and also reduces cholesterol in the blood. All pungent spices, including ginger, cloves, horseradish, and mustard, open the peripheral blood vessels, encourage sweating, and, in moderation, can be helpful to the circulation. Herbs such as rosemary, thyme, bay, mint, and sage all have useful medicinal effects. They are anti-infective, they are antioxidants that preserve beneficial body fats, and they are helpful for stomach and intestinal problems.

The old adage "you are what you eat" applies most of all to fats and oils. Studies have shown that the oils we eat become an integral part of the membranes of our cells and the lining of our arteries and veins. We have already mentioned the value of minimizing your fat intake. However, it is worth remembering that there are essential oils that can help our circulation and general health and reduce cholesterol. EPA in fish oil and the oils in some nuts have been shown to lower cholesterol levels.

Purslane is a salad plant used in Crete, which, like walnuts, has a high level of alpha-linoleic acid, one of the essential oils we need to make hormones and other substances. The Cretans have one of the lowest levels of heart disease in the world. In the recent Lyon Heart Study, based at Lyon, France, 606 people who had already suffered heart attacks were divided into two groups. Half were put on the traditional Cretan diet, which included rough bread, salads, olive oil, feta cheese, and purslane, and the other half were put on the low-cholesterol diet recommended by the American Heart Association. Those on the Cretan diet did much better and incurred far fewer subsequent heart attacks than the other group. The experiment was stopped after two years because it was judged unethical to continue to deny the second group the most effective dietary recommendations.

OTHER HERBS AND SUPPLEMENTS
FOR THE CIRCULATION

Though garlic is uniquely effective as a daily preventive remedy for the circulation, there are other herbs and food supplements that are of special interest.

Fish Oil, Containing EPA

EPA is a fat that is made by the human body in small amounts. It is a starting material for the manufacture of prostaglandins, which influence clotting and local constriction of the blood vessels. It is able to reduce platelet clumping, increase clotting time, and improve the blood's fat content. As a result of many clinical studies around the world, fish oil containing EPA is now accepted as a medicine by health authorities. Besides being available on pharmacy shelves, it is also given as a prescription for patients with heart disease.

The clinical studies have almost all been done on the main fish oil product, which is called MaxEPA. This has been shown to relieve angina and peripheral vascular disease. It lowers the levels of cholesterol and blood fat, especially that of one of the main carriers of cholesterol, very-low-density lipoprotein. It also reduces clotting and stickiness. Fish oils are a nutritional supplement which, in the long run, will gradually adjust the fat content in the tissues. Garlic is more medicinal and works more immediately than EPA, although its effects wear off more quickly when it is not taken. Garlic seems to reduce cholesterol and LDL more markedly than EPA, but to have a different effect on the clotting process, which is more connected to platelets and clot-dissolving effects, rather than the effects on local hormones that reduce clotting— the prostaglandins. Garlic and EPA therefore make good partners, complementing each other by working differently against the buildup of atherosclerosis.

Magnesium and Other Minerals

Magnesium is the mineral most closely linked to heart problems. Many experts believe that a lack of magnesium in the diet produces heart damage, sensitivity of the heart to attack by stress hormones, and problems with heart rhythm. A lack of magnesium may be a cause of sudden death in people with heart disease. It can protect the heart during and after a heart attack. It would be wise to take magnesium if there is a magnesium deficiency in the diet. The recommended level is 300 mg a day, and a processed-food diet may contain only a fraction of this. Dark green vegetables, nuts, seeds, whole meal flour, and molasses are all rich in magnesium. The presence of magnesium in the water supply may be the reason for the lower levels of heart disease in areas which have hard water, compared to those with soft. There are also some other minerals which are needed in small amounts for a healthy circulation, including zinc, copper, and selenium. A varied natural diet will normally provide the levels required.

Vitamin E

Vitamin E is a somewhat mysterious fatty vitamin. It has had a controversial past, with many scientists doubting that it was indeed a vitamin. However, it is now becoming clear that together with vitamin C and selenium, it is part of the body's antioxidation system. This ensures that the body fats do not become rancid, and helps to protect the walls of the arteries and the blood cells. For that reason, vitamin E can be used to treat diseases of the peripheral circulation, for example, in the legs or the eyes. It helps to move oxygen around the body, and can bring extra amounts to the heart and protect it from damage during atherosclerosis. If you are vulnerable to heart disease or have raised blood cholesterol, it might be worthwhile to take supplements of vitamin E. However, since sudden, large doses can raise blood pressure, it is best to take vitamin E under the guidance of a medical or nutritional expert. Small amounts of vitamin E are available in wheat germ and in whole grains.

Rutin

Rutin is a material that is found in the flowers and leaves of buckwheat. It protects fragile blood vessels. For that reason, it is used to prevent damage to the small blood vessels and as a treatment of varicose veins. It is available only as a supplement. If rutin is unavailable, both bilberries (blueberries) and rosemary can be used as a substitute, since both these plants contain capillary-protecting ingredients. Bilberries can be taken as a food and rosemary as an herb tea.

Herbal Medicines for the Heart

There are a range of herbal medicines that are used to treat heart conditions, either as a replacement for, or in addition to, conventional medical treatment. The herbalist can often provide mixtures that are effective at an early stage of heart disease, when the use of conventional drugs is rejected because of side effects. All these herbs should be used under professional guidance for proper effect. Possibilities include:

- *Hawthorn (Crataegus oxyacantha)*, particularly the flowers and leaves, is one of the main remedies for the heart, stimulating circulation in the coronary vessels and protecting and supporting the heart muscle in old age and heart disease.

- *Ginkgo biloba* is an ancient Oriental remedy that has recently been rediscovered. It opens the arteries and therefore helps the peripheral circulation and the circulation in the brain.

- *Mistletoe (Viscum album)* can be used for high blood pressure and is effective over long periods. It helps with symptoms such as dizziness. It should be used only under professional guidance.

- *Butcher's broom (Ruscus aculeatus)* is a root used to restore circulation in the veins rather than the arteries. It is used to treat varicose veins and is a diuretic, removing excess water from the body. The flowers of broom have a special heart-supporting effect; they regulate the heart-beat and help prevent disturbances of heart rhythm.

- *Lily of the Valley (Convallaria majalis)* is a heart stimulant and will help to support a weak heart.

Special Fiber-Containing Herbs to Reduce Cholesterol

There are certain fiber-containing herbs that clean out excess cholesterol in the form of bile, and therefore have significant cholesterol-lowering effects. They work similarly to the fibrate type of mild cholesterol-lowering drugs, and are at least as effective. These are alfalfa seed, linseed, psyllium seed, and especially fenugreek seed, all of which can be taken in food as powders. There have been many studies on these seeds. For example, one study by Dr. Jorgen Molgaard and colleagues reported in the journal *Atherosclerosis* showed that alfalfa seed could lower cholesterol up to 25 percent in a group of patients with high levels of blood fats.

DAILY HEART CARE—AN OVERVIEW

We have looked at a number of aspects of our daily lives. Poor diet, too much salt, lack of exercise, stress, toxins, and smoking (see inset on next page) have been identified scientifically as the main causes of atherosclerosis and heart disease. Garlic, EPA, magnesium, fiber, and herbs offer positive protection. But how are we to remember all this advice? It must, at times, seem complex enough to make us throw up our hands, order a good steak, and say, "To hell with health!" The solution is to keep recalling the reason why there is an epidemic of heart disease. Remember that it is a new event; our ancestors were not affected by it. Nor are the so-called primitive peoples, the aborigines, the Bedouin, the Zulus, or the Eskimos, even if they eat meat and smoke. Animals, too, don't suffer from heart disease unless we experimentally feed them our own diets.

The main reason for the epidemic is that the modern world has relentlessly substituted synthetic products and materials for the real thing. Wild animals grazing on wild plants produce meat that contains EPA and a minimum of

SMOKING

Smokers have a much higher risk of heart disease. This is partly because nicotine constricts the blood vessels, especially the coronary arteries. The carbon monoxide from the burning tobacco also puts a strain on the heart. Nicotine is probably the most widely used toxin in our society, and giving up smoking is not easy. There is, nevertheless, a steady social move away from it, which should be helpful. Probably the best thing to do is to spend as much time as possible with nonsmokers. Try to add other things to your life to take its place—whether an interest or hobby, a walk, or nibbling some nuts and raisins. Most people put on weight after giving up cigarettes, but this can be dealt with when it happens.

saturated fat. Vegetables and whole grains have always been full of minerals and necessary nutrients. Instead, we have processed them mercilessly. Exercise was once a natural part of daily life. Now we are obliged to sit around all week and confine ourselves to unhealthy bursts carried out, if at all, on weekends. Stress used to be reserved for special events. Now it is relaxation that is special. Garlic and other medicines used to be everyday foods, built into the diet through the natural wisdom of society. Now we have to write books about their health benefits in order to persuade people to go back to them.

The logic of the do's and don'ts is to keep as much as possible to the simpler and more tangible aspects of life. When in doubt, select the more unrefined, the more substantial, the less artificial. It may not be so convenient to cook fresh vegetables. But then, a heart attack is not convenient, either.

There is another essential guide, and that is yourself. You may not feel atherosclerosis creeping up. But if you do take care of yourself in the ways outlined above, you will feel better, more positive, more energetic, and have fewer petty symptoms. Exercise will make you feel good. Vegetarian food will make you feel lighter. Relaxation will help you perform better.

CHAPTER 8

Garlic's Other Actions

Although scientists today are mostly concerned with garlic's actions on the circulation, garlic is also famous for its treatment of infections. It is perhaps more well-known in herbal history for this use than any other, because as a leading herbal antibiotic, it must have saved many lives. Before the discovery of the first antibacterial drugs—Salvarsan and sulfonamides—in the early twentieth century, garlic's own sulfurs were commonly used as "the people's antibiotic" in a tradition stretching back to ancient times. In Eastern Europe, Russia, and elsewhere, this has continued to the present day, and there is now renewed interest everywhere in garlic's anti-infective properties. In this chapter, we will examine some of the ways in which garlic helps to fight infections.

THE TREATMENT OF INFECTIONS

Garlic does not act against bacteria as powerfully or as

precisely as modern antibiotics; it is slower and somewhat weaker. However, it does not have the side effects that antibiotics do. Nor has it been known to create bacterial resistance; in laboratory tests, bacteria have never become so accustomed to garlic that they could survive with it, or even survive on it, as happens frequently with modern drugs. Its other main advantage is that it is able to act against a very wide range of bacteria.

Its main use is therefore in infections that are not acute or immediately life-threatening. One would not use garlic against pneumonia, for example, or a runaway leg infection, or acute dysentery. It deals best with chronic and less dangerous infections, such as sore throats, laryngitis, bronchitis, catarrh, sinusitis, gum infections, coughs, diarrhea, indigestion, mild gastroenteritis, cystitis, skin infections, boils, and so on. In such cases, the only solution offered by conventional, modern medicine—antibiotics—may not be worth the cost in side effects. Moreover, some of these infections tend to recur and require repeated doses of antibiotics, which, over time, may make the side effects more serious and even encourage recurrences. Garlic is a milder, safer, and no less effective substitute.

In the case of fungal and yeast infections, the situation is even more in garlic's favor. These are often treated by medical drugs that take some time to work, and can create even more side effects than antibiotics. Drugs used against ringworm and other prolonged fungal skin infections can inhibit the white blood cells, and in many cases work more slowly than an active treatment with garlic. Fungal infections tend to be nagging and continuous rather than fast and dangerous, and so are very suitable for garlic's more gentle, persistent action. As we shall see, there is evidence that garlic may be just as strong as the usual antifungal drugs, and very wide in its field of action.

Fungal and yeast problems suitable for treatment by garlic include ringworm, athlete's foot, cystitis, thrush, vaginitis, and *Candida* infections; all are particularly irritating and hard to eliminate by modern medicine. *Candida*, in particular, is a very widespread and ever-increasing health problem. Like other fungal infections, it tends to recur because the previous use of antibiotics and steroids has harmed the body's immunity. It has been suggested that a whole range of health problems result from *Candida* infections, particularly in the intestine. These include allergies (since *Candida* may damage the intestine, allowing allergy-causing materials to leak through), fatigue and debility, and blood sugar problems. Garlic is the ideal remedy, and is frequently prescribed by naturopathic doctors treating these problems.

In the treatment of infections, whether fungal or bacterial, garlic should be used quite aggressively. The dose should be substantial—it is necessary to take several cloves a day for real anti-infective action. However, garlic should not be left to work alone, especially in dealing with more persistent problems. Garlic should not be regarded as just another antibiotic, albeit one somewhat closer to nature. It should be used in a holistic way, combined with nutritional and other self-care measures. The basic anti-infective regimen involves fasting. This need not be complete, however; eating only fruit and green salads for a few days will give a powerful boost to the immune system and help towards a complete cure. Along with fasting, it is useful to take drinks of hot lemon juice, preferably with 1 teaspoonful of grated fresh ginger, hot cider vinegar with honey, and some vitamin C. These drinks help to clean out toxins and speed the immune components through the body. My own family uses this kind of regimen whenever we have an infection, and none of us have needed antibiotics for thirteen years.

THE EVIDENCE

There is a great deal of scientific evidence for garlic's anti-infective power. Its extent is far greater than most people realize. The first person to demonstrate it was the famous Louis Pasteur, in 1858. He grew a covering of bacteria in a laboratory culture dish; when he dropped garlic juice into the dish, it killed all the bacteria around it. This kind of experiment has been repeated continuously over the years on both bacteria and yeasts, and the number of these experiments has recently been increasing with the new awareness of the need for safe medicines from plants.

A study carried out at the University of Londrina in Brazil in 1982 showed that garlic juice was highly effective against twenty-one kinds of bacteria which cause stomach problems, including *Salmonella, Proteus, Shigella* (the organism which causes dysentery), and coliforms. Garlic juice stopped the growth of the bacteria as effectively as ampicillin. A study at the University of California at Davis showed that a 1 to 20 dilution of dried garlic in water could kill *Salmonella* speedily; after one hour, only 10 percent of the bacteria survived, and after another hour this was down to one percent. The scientists tried and failed to find evidence of bacteria that had become resistant to garlic.

Salmonella infections in food affect millions of people annually. Garlic is an obvious recourse. If it were included in the diet, it would help to prevent any *Salmonella* present from causing a stomach infection in the first place. In most cases, stomach infections are mild and not dangerous, so garlic would be the ideal treatment, rather than stronger, modern drugs. In addition, garlic appears to be more effective at killing the infective bacteria, rather than those that normally live in the intestine.

Laboratory studies have shown that a very wide range of bacteria is sensitive to garlic, and that the range is wider than that of commonly used antibiotics. The bacteria that cause throat, mouth, stomach, skin, lung, and other infections are particularly sensitive, as are those that cause food poisoning. Garlic also kills bacteria that have become resistant to other antibiotics. However, if a specific amount of garlic juice is placed in the middle of a dish of bacteria, and its effect compared to that of a similar amount of a modern antibiotic such as penicillin, tetracycline, or erythromycin, it is weaker. Various studies have put the power of garlic at about 1 to 10 percent of these other antibiotics.

Although there are many fascinating early medical reports on the success of garlic, even against such intractable infections as tuberculosis, there are not, at present, any modern clinical research studies of the treatment of bacterial diseases in humans. Intriguing doctors' reports do exist, however, documenting the successful use of garlic to treat dysentery and other digestive problems, as well as infected wounds, by military doctors during the First and Second World Wars.

There is also a great deal of scientific evidence concerning the wide range of garlic's antifungal effects. Laboratory studies have demonstrated that it can kill organisms such as *Aspergillus, Cryptococcus, Penicillium, Microsporum, Candida,* and *Histoplasma*. In this case, garlic is as strong as regular, modern drugs, besides being a great deal safer. A classic study of the effect of garlic on *Candida* was carried out by Dr. Frank Barone and Dr. Michael Tansey of the University of Indiana. They showed that the amount of garlic needed to kill *Candida* was the same as that of modern treatments, for example, a 3 percent lotion of amphotericin B for external use and 1 g of griseofulvin taken internally. Other reports suggest that fresh garlic is stronger against *Candida* than nystatin.

There have been some preliminary studies on the use of garlic in fungal infections, especially in animals. *Candida* infections were cured experimentally in chickens by adding garlic to their diet. The growth of ringworm and other skin fungal infections in rabbits was stopped immediately by putting garlic on the infection; this healed within fourteen days, at least as rapidly as would be expected with the modern drugs which would normally be used. (However, garlic had no effect on the infections when given to the rabbits in their diet.) Its ability to control all kinds of infections in livestock animals has long been noticed by farmers and animal breeders, and its veterinary use has quite a following today.

There is a certain amount of evidence for garlic's antifungal effects in humans, as well. For example, a study was carried out at the Veterans Administration Medical Center in East Orange, New Jersey, in which the juice of 10 g of garlic (three cloves) was given to volunteers. After half an hour, their blood serum was able to kill *Candida*. This effect did not pass into the urine. An interesting observation appeared in the *Medical Journal of Australia*, submitted by a doctor who had treated a member of his own family for ringworm on the arms. In the interests of science, he treated one arm with garlic and the other with an antifungal drug. The garlic-treated arm healed in ten days, while the other took twice as long.

It is very clear which active ingredient of garlic principally achieves these antibacterial and antifungal effects: it is allicin, which is present in fresh garlic. Garlic oil has proved not to be as strong when tested in the laboratory.

THE EFFECT OF GARLIC ON WORMS AND PARASITES

The use of garlic against worms and parasites also has a long history, and has been mentioned in the very earliest records. This is an extension of its effect on bacteria and yeasts, since results are achieved in the same way: the reactive sulfur compounds attack the organisms invading the body, but are not dangerous to body tissue.

Garlic is recommended against pinworms or thread-worms, and can be taken in through both ends of the digestive system. After eating garlic or using it as a suppository, large numbers of worms are excreted. Parasites that live higher up in the digestive system are also affected by it, but a longer-term persistence may be necessary in order to dislodge them.

Interestingly, garlic has recently been shown to be very effective in killing the organism that produces amoebic dysentery; it is as effective as metronidazole, the main drug currently used, at least in the laboratory. Professor David Mirelman, of the Department of Parasitology at the Weizman Institute in Israel, believes that garlic could one day benefit the millions of amoebic dysentery sufferers around the world, not only because it has fewer side effects than regular, modern drugs, but also because it is cheap and can be grown locally. (See *Garlic in the Garden* inset on page 100.)

GARLIC CAN REDUCE BLOOD SUGAR

If animals are fed garlic and then given a lot of sugar, the amount of sugar in their blood falls far short of the expected peak. Garlic is able to reduce blood sugar levels and encourage the process that takes up the sugar in the blood and turns it into carbohydrates in the liver. It has been found that garlic increases the amount of insulin, which is in charge of gathering up excess sugar. This has been studied by giving garlic to animals with mild diabetes; the production of insulin was stimulated and sugar levels

GARLIC IN THE GARDEN

Bearing in mind that many readers will take the health of their gardens very much to heart, a few comments on the use of garlic against pests, worms, and fungi in the garden would be appropriate although it is, strictly, outside our theme.

The farmers of old used to plant garlic near their onions, cabbages, and other vegetables because it kept away various flies and grubs. Modern organic gardeners have found that garlic extract, highly diluted, kills or keeps away wireworms, caterpillars, weevils, and blackflies. The key to making a good garden concoction is to crush the garlic, leave it to generate its oily sulfides, and then dilute it with water and oil-based soap. The active insect-killing materials are the sulfides in the oil, and these are quite strong. Studies at the University of California have shown that mosquito larvae are killed by a dilution of one crushed clove in four liters of water.

Garlic is as useful against the fungi in the garden as it is in the body. Try it against mildew, beam rust, anthracnose, brown rot, and blight.

were reduced by around 20 percent, an effect equivalent to that of the antidiabetic drug tolbutamide. In this case, the effect of onion is equivalent to, or even greater than, that of garlic.

This does not make garlic a cure for diabetes. However, it might encourage people with prediabetes or poor sugar metabolism to try garlic as a useful supplement to the diet.

GARLIC AS A PROTECTION AGAINST CANCER AND POISONS

The sulfur compounds in garlic are not unlike those in the body that act as the first defense against poisons. The liver uses such compounds to detoxify and disintegrate drugs, poisons, and unwanted body chemicals. In 1953, Dr. A.S. Weissberger of Case Western University in Cleveland, Ohio, suggested that the sulfur in allicin might also protect against cancer by helping to remove cancer cells. He injected cancer cells into mice with or without a small amount of allicin from garlic. The mice who were injected with the cancer alone lived for only sixteen days, the others for six months.

This awakened some interest in the possibility of garlic as a preventive against cancer. Professor Sydney Belman of the New York Medical Center found that onion and garlic oil were both able to prevent much of the expected cancer in mice injected with cancer-causing chemicals. Professor Michael Wargovich of the Department of Medical Oncology at the M.D. Anderson Hospital in Houston, Texas, recently found that he could prevent three-quarters of the expected, chemically-caused tumors by giving mice diallyl sulfide, one of the group of sulfides that make up garlic oil.

Well over a hundred of these kinds of studies have now been carried out, involving cells, animals, and tissues, and it is quite clear that garlic, garlic oil, allicin, the sulfides, and most garlic compounds are effective in protecting against almost every kind of cancer, and can also protect against genetic changes in the DNA. However, it should be stressed that garlic seems to be a cancer preventive, not a cancer cure—there is no evidence that it can help to treat any cancer, and it would be most unwise to rely on garlic for this purpose.

In Third World countries, the folk tradition often regards

garlic and onion as cancer preventives. For example, in China, garlic and green tea are both thought of as protective against stomach and lung cancer. The evidence from animal studies has sufficed to interest the National Cancer Institute in Bethesda, Maryland, which began a $20 million "designer foods" research program to see if adding components found in specific foods to the diet would help reduce the risk of cancer. Garlic was one of the food items selected for research, along with rosemary, licorice, and several more. There is no direct evidence that garlic acts as a cancer preventive in people; however, there are several studies showing that people who live in garlic-eating areas seem to incur fewer cancers. An intriguing observation comes from China. Dr. Xing Mei of Shandong Medical College observed that the people of Gangshan County had stomach cancer rates of 3.5 per 100,000 people. In the neighboring Qixia County, the stomach cancer rates were more than ten times higher, at 40 per 100,000 people. The only thing he could find to account for the difference was that the people of Gangshan each ate on average about six cloves of garlic a day, and those from Qixia ate none. Another example is an American study published in 1994 by Dr. K. Steinmetz and colleagues called the Iowa Women's Health Study. The intake of 127 separate foods was monitored in 41,387 women. Of all the foods eaten, only garlic was clearly associated with a reduced risk of colon cancer.

Garlic's sulfur groups are also able to gather up toxic heavy metals in the body. The use of sulfur compounds for this purpose is well known in medicine. Indeed, one of the conventional treatments used in hospitals for heavy metal poisoning is to give cysteine, which is a sulfur-containing amino acid similar to alliin. In Bulgaria, a garlic preparation called Satal was used to help workers overcome industrial lead poisoning; it greatly reduced the symptoms of the poisoning and the amounts of heavy metals in the blood. Garlic can capture nearly its own weight of lead or mercury and, once bound, these metals can be eliminated. A number of laboratory studies with animals have showed that garlic can speed up the elimination of heavy metals as powerfully as conventional drugs used for this purpose. It can also help to clean out other substances, such as food additives or solvents.

In the past, people were much more concerned about infections than they were about heart disease, for heart disease was a rarity, but infections were a daily threat which could be lethal. Garlic was one of the main weapons against such infections, able to kill the bacteria or fungi, and also detoxify the body. As nature's main antibiotic, it was regarded with the greatest respect until the invention of chemical antibiotics. Today, though we do not need to turn the clock back and rely on garlic exclusively, we nevertheless can use and appreciate garlic for a wide range of minor infections. The chemical antibiotics have their role to play for more serious or acute problems, but garlic should still take pride of place in our kitchen pharmacy.

CHAPTER 9

Garlic Products and Preparations

arlic is as effective a medicine as some modern drugs. It can thin the blood as efficiently as the other favorite, a little aspirin every day. It can reduce the buildup of fats in the circulation as well as, or better than, cholestyramine, a drug often used for this purpose that is not completely safe, since it can cause a variety of digestive side effects. Garlic's anti-infective properties may be nearly as good as those of the modern antifungal drugs. Garlic, however, is different in that it is a plant and a natural medicinal food. It is not a pill containing a precise amount of pure chemicals, to be swallowed unthinkingly twice a day. It requires more attention from you. It is important to understand the different garlic products available, so that you can choose the one that best suits you. You will need to know how much to take, and the most effective way of taking it for your particular purposes. According to your own preferences, you will also need to know the various ways of reducing the smell. This sounds a lot to take in, but perhaps one should apply the same kind of consideration to any plant, whether it is used as a food or a medicine. To get the best from garlic, get involved with it. You will find a special fun in knowing your subject thoroughly, and your cooking will benefit too.

HOW MUCH TO TAKE

When taking garlic, there are three levels of dosage you should be aware of.

"Preventive" Dose

For all preventive purposes, including the protection of the circulation, you should take at least one clove of garlic, weighing from 2 to 3 grams, a day. This is the minimum, or preventive, dose. It is advisable to split the dose, as studies have shown that garlic stays in the body for just a few hours before it is removed or neutralized. Therefore, it is necessary to take at least one to one and a half grams (or half a clove) morning and evening.

"Therapeutic" Dose

There are situations where you will need to take much more than the preventive dose. When you use garlic to treat an illness or a symptom—bronchial and throat problems, *Candida,* stomach infections, skin infections, and so on—then a larger, therapeutic dose is required. The reason is that you need a much more powerful punch to knock out bacteria, yeasts, or fungi than to inhibit cholesterol, fats, and blood clots in the circulation. The therapeutic dose should be a minimum of one clove's worth (2 to 3 g) three times a day. This is the amount suggested by the British herbal pharmacopoeia, traditional sources, and modern herbal guides. In my own experience, it is the minimum needed to maintain a real antiseptic and antibiotic action in the body tissues. For those who rarely touch garlic, this dose may seem like a lot. However, it is really not so large a dose; in many societies—in parts of China, for example—people would eat this much or more on a regular basis, children included.

The therapeutic dose is not normally required in order to take care of your circulation, although occasionally it may be advisable to take this dose. If you have had or are having a very heavy or fatty meal, or if you suspect the wholesomeness of the food, it would be worth neutralizing it with one or two cloves of garlic. Again, in more serious cases of circulatory disease or atherosclerosis, garlic may be used at a higher dose as part of a therapeutic program in order to regain health.

"Saturation" Dose

Very occasionally, and unusually, it may be necessary to take very large doses indeed—a whole head of garlic or more. This is what we would call a saturation dose. This would occur where more serious infections, such as abscesses, dysentery, or septic wounds, were developing and you were unable or unwilling to take modern drugs. You should obtain professional advice in such cases, anyway.

TAKING FRESH GARLIC

Fresh garlic should be taken either with a quantity of warm water or milk, with fruit such as apples and pears, with vegetable juices or soups, or with green salads such as lettuce and parsley. All of these methods will help to eliminate the burning sensation in the mouth or stomach.

Green leafy vegetables, especially parsley, will also reduce the subsequent familiar aroma.

Fresh garlic is still medicinally effective if eaten with food. However, the body may not be able to absorb all the garlic if it is taken with a full meal, so in such a case it is advisable to increase the amount. Here are some more detailed ways of taking fresh garlic that you might like to try:

- *Garlic in milk or yogurt.* Crush one clove in half a cup of warm milk (goat's milk if preferred). Add honey to taste. This is an old gypsy remedy. Since milk is not the best drink to take when there are chest or throat infections, or where there is mucus, this remedy can be modified by substituting kumiss or yogurt.

- *Garlic syrup.* This is similar to the garlic syrups described in the official drug guides, such as the British pharmacopoeia, in the early twentieth century. It is recommended by many herbalists as a handy and effective item to keep in your medicine chest, ready when needed. The garlic is not fresh, as in the other recipes, and some of the allicin will have decayed, but it seems to keep its power remarkably well. Put 250 g (about ten heads or eighty cloves) of crushed garlic in a 1-liter jar. Almost fill with cider vinegar and water in equal amounts, cover and leave for a few days, shaking occasionally. Strain through a cloth, add 1 cup of honey, stir, and keep in the refrigerator. This syrup will keep for up to a year. It is especially useful for coughs, nasal and bronchial problems, and sore throats, as well as for circulatory problems. One tablespoon three times a day is the correct dose.

- *Garlic and miso soup.* Miso, a Japanese soybean extract, makes an excellent hot soup, ideal to take with garlic.

Dissolve a teaspoonful of miso in just-boiled water. Add a couple of drops of soy sauce, a good squeeze of lemon, some grated onion, and one or two crushed cloves of garlic. This is especially good during the convalescent period of an infection, as it brings strength as well as healing. In a pinch, a concentrated vegetable stock can be substituted for the miso.

- *External applications of fresh garlic.* There are situations—for example, athlete's foot, fungal infections, stings, *Candida* in the urogenital area, or tooth and gum infections—where garlic needs to be applied directly to the skin or mucosal surfaces. If the skin is not overly sensitive, one can simply crush garlic onto a small piece of cotton, place it on the area, and bind it. There may be some burning sensation, which passes in a few minutes. The garlic can be kept to the required area by spreading petroleum jelly on the surrounding parts. If the burning would otherwise be too intense, for example, on the gums, one can use a slice of garlic which has been left for thirty minutes after crushing.

HOW TO DEAL WITH THE ODOR

Garlic's strong odor comes mostly from the sulfides and disulfides which are formed by the natural changes in the allicin. When you eat fresh garlic, the immediate odor arises from the mouth and the teeth; some more comes from the stomach, and the rest from the lungs and skin. You can substantially reduce the mouth odor by swallowing ready-crushed garlic quickly without chewing it, by washing it down with liquid, or by making a "pill" with lettuce or parsley. Once, I suggested to my youngest daughter, when she was around 5 years old, that she take garlic for a minor infection. Later that morning, I happened to see her concentrating intensely on something in the kitchen. I peeped over her shoulder, and found her cutting peeled garlic cloves into slivers, inserting them into grapes, and eating them gleefully. What a delightful way she had discovered of taking her medicine! Lettuce, parsley, and aromatic seeds such as anise seed, mint, and cloves all reduce and disguise the odors from the stomach. These should be eaten with, and after, the garlic. The odor from the skin and lungs cannot be avoided, but it is milder. However, if the odor is a problem, the best way to reduce it is undoubtedly to use one of the other garlic products available on the market (see below). Some of these employ very interesting modern methods to reduce and virtually eliminate the odor.

FRIED AND COOKED GARLIC

If garlic is crushed in a frying pan, some allicin is produced immediately, and then the heat of the cooking converts it to the oily and strongly odorous sulfides and disulfides. As we have seen, these compounds are effective in cardiovascular protection, so frying or cooking garlic does not destroy its effectiveness. On the other hand, these sulfur compounds do gradually vaporize into the air, and so are lost. When your neighbor smells the garlicky aromas coming from your kitchen, it means that your garlic dish has lost some of its medicinal compounds. So, you should only add garlic at the end of the cooking time, and remember that after the process, the amount of garlic you may actually be getting in your plate might be small.

GARLIC PRODUCTS

As we have seen, garlic products have become extremely popular in the last few years. They provide an opportunity to share in the undoubted health benefits of garlic without any of the admittedly mild side effects. Their main popularity has been in Northern Europe and in the United States, where garlic is not yet a national flavor. There are many garlic products, from the comparatively odorous to the completely deodorized. These come in the form of oils, powders, extracts, pills, and capsules. How effective are they? Which ones are best? The products are divided into three main groups.

Garlic Oil Capsules

Garlic oil is the essential or aromatic oil of garlic. It is made by mashing garlic in a vat, and then bubbling steam through it. The oily components are carried through on the steam, and then collected once the steam has cooled.

Another way of making garlic oil is to add a large quantity of vegetable oil to mashed garlic in a vat, without heating it. The vegetable oil takes up the garlic oil, after which the solids are removed by filtration. This is called an oil macerate and is used in some European oil capsules.

The oil of garlic is made up of sulfides, disulfides, trisulfides, and other compounds that are formed from the transformation of allicin. In ordinary fresh garlic, or in fresh garlic mixed with vegetable oil, this change happens over a few days. When mashed garlic is steam-distilled, this happens immediately because of the heat, as it does when garlic is fried. Garlic oil is therefore very similar to fried garlic. The amount of the oil is roughly the same as the amount of allicin which produced it, that is, from 0.1 to 0.2 percent of the total weight. In other words, at least 500 to 1,000 kg of fresh garlic gives 1 kg of oil. This makes it extremely concentrated. One clove weighing 2 to 3 grams would contain 2 to 6 milligrams (or thousandths of a gram) of the oil.

Garlic oil is normally sold in capsules, in which a very

small amount is suspended in vegetable oil and enclosed in gelatin. These capsules were the very first of the garlic products, developed in the 1920s in Germany, and they have been consistently popular ever since. In fact, most of the 300 million doses of garlic consumed in the United Kingdom in 1995 were in the form of garlic oil capsules. Garlic capsules completely avoid the mouth odor that comes from chewing garlic; however, the contents themselves have a strong garlic odor that can emerge on the breath after the capsules are dissolved in the stomach. The odor can be reduced even further by "enteric coating," in which the capsules are coated with a substance that prevents them from dissolving in the stomach. Instead, they pass through it and dissolve in the intestine, thus avoiding the odor and burping that sometimes occurs with ordinary capsules.

But are these capsules effective? There have been a number of studies on this question. It has been found by scientists like Professor Arun Bordia, a pioneer of garlic research in India, and Dr. Asat Qureshi, of the United States Department of Agriculture, that the oil is as effective as fresh garlic at reducing cholesterol and blood clotting, and as a general cardiovascular preventive. Thus, the popularity of garlic capsules over the years has been confirmed in the laboratory. However, the antibiotic potency of garlic oil capsules is limited. Studies have shown that fresh garlic or garlic juice which is placed in the middle of a "sea" of bacteria will kill all those within a distance of several centimeters. If garlic oil is used, the power to kill the bacteria or fungi is much reduced, though it is still present.

We have seen that one clove of garlic will produce 2 to 6 mg of oil. This is a daily "preventive" dose. Many capsules on the market today contain less than 1 mg of oil, often only 0.66 mg. The reason, in part, is that this is the traditional dosage, set in the dim and distant past. One will need two to nine such capsules per day to achieve the minimum preventive dose, and six to twenty-seven capsules per day to achieve the therapeutic dose corresponding to three cloves.

In fact, a number of researchers, such as Dr. R.R. Samson of the Edinburgh Royal Infirmary, have carried out studies on patients using the oil capsules. It turned out that when oil that is freshly prepared in the laboratory is used, the thinning of the blood and the reducing of cholesterol can be clearly demonstrated. But when some oil capsules were used according to the manufacturers' recommendations, no results were obtained. These oil capsules failed through inadequate dosage. So, make sure that there is sufficient dosage in the capsules you are considering; the package should tell you how much garlic oil the capsules contain, in addition to the filler, which is usually vegetable oil.

Dried Garlic Powder Tablets

Another way of concentrating garlic and making it into a pharmaceutical product is by drying it. Garlic is nearly two-thirds water, so drying it produces a powder which is then ready to put into tablets. These tablets can then be coated to reduce the aroma. This is a potentially good way of preserving the medicinal qualities of garlic, since it is possible to achieve high levels of allicin in such powders. The garlic powder tablets are very popular, and most of the clinical trials on reducing cholesterol have used this kind of product. These tablets can be virtually odor-free; in the clinical study already mentioned by Dr. F.H. Mader and colleagues, only about 10 percent of the participants noticed an odor.

The drying process sounds very simple, but is in fact very complicated. Special conditions are necessary in order to produce the maximum amounts of allicin and active ingredients in the dried powder. For example, if the garlic is ground and dried very quickly, there will be no time for it to make allicin; you will get a more or less odorless and less effective powder. On the other hand, if it is prepared slowly, the allicin will alter spontaneously to produce the oily compounds, and the powder will have a strong smell.

This is the case with the dried garlic used in food. The food industry dries a great deal of garlic into powder, flakes, and granules. The drying process uses higher temperatures and longer times, compared to when garlic is dried for medicinal use, with the result that the allicin is lost. Even the oil content is minimal, due to processing and long storage. For these reasons, the dried garlic powder or granules you find in the supermarket are not suitable as a medicine.

Due to the different methods of drying garlic, the powders can therefore vary from very good to very poor. This presents a problem for the consumer, who has a right to know the potency of any product. Fortunately, there are two tests which can be done to assess whether or not the powder contains high levels of allicin. One you can do yourself, the other must be done by the manufacturer.

- *The taste test.* Allicin is pungent and burning, but it does not have a heavy odor. The oily sulfides that are produced from allicin, on the other hand, have the typically rich, heavy, clinging, sulfurous aroma of garlic, but do not have a burning taste. So, you can test the contents of a pill or capsule by taste. First, it should be strong, otherwise it will be no good at all. Second, it should have both the burning taste of allicin (the more the better) and the rich aroma of the sulfides.

- *The analytic test.* It is now possible to analyze garlic extracts and products by a technique called High Pressure Liquid Chromatography (HPLC). This will tell the chemist exactly how much alliin and allicin a product contains, and how much of the other components. Manufacturers should state the content of allicin and other components of their garlic powder tablets on the packaging.

If the powder is well-made, it should be equally effective for the protection of the circulation and in the other areas where garlic is useful. This is an area of active research. In China, Europe, and the United States, efforts are being made to produce the perfect garlic powder extract for medicinal use.

Deodorized "Aged" Garlic

The third type of garlic product that you might encounter in the health-food stores is an extract, made in Japan, that is described as deodorized. It is made by chopping garlic and aging it in alcohol over many months. An extract is made from this, which is then used as the basis for tablets and other preparations. The aged garlic preparations appear to have a somewhat different chemical profile from the other garlic preparations, and are not based on the creation of allicin or the sulfide substances derived from it. The lack of odor is due to the lack of these odorous components rather than the special ways in which they are packed, which is how the odor is dealt with in the other products.

There is quite a lot of debate in the health product industry and the scientific literature concerning the effectiveness of deodorized, as compared to regular, garlic products. The situation is unclear, especially because there have never been clinical studies in which the effectiveness of different forms of garlic has been compared. The lack of such studies means that this debate is based on inference. Deodorized garlic appears to lack certain key active ingredients that act on the circulation, but it does have others that have anticancer effects. Though the different forms of garlic have not been compared clinically, one can say with certainty that the vast majority of clinical and scientific research on garlic powder tablets and garlic oil capsules show their effectiveness in the cardiovascular area, while the majority of studies on the aged deodorized garlic show its effectiveness in the cancer preventive area discussed in Chapter 8.

THE SAFETY OF GARLIC AND GARLIC PRODUCTS

Garlic is extremely safe, and is consumed by millions of people daily all over the world, without adverse effects. There are groups of people whose traditional foods include several cloves a day of fresh garlic, without any signs of harm. For example, the people of Gangshan County in Shandong Province, China, consume about 20 grams of fresh garlic a day—about seven cloves. In some studies on cholesterol reduction, up to twenty cloves of fresh garlic a day were given for three months, without ill effects. People have taken 200 milligrams of garlic oil—equivalent to seventy cloves of garlic—without ill effects.

Garlic can only be toxic at impossibly high doses. Studies in rats have shown that toxic effects occurred at a dose of 5 grams of fresh juice per kilogram of body weight, which is equivalent to a man eating 300 mashed cloves in one sitting. At this kind of dose, the stomach can be injured by the pungency of fresh garlic, as it would by other pungent substances such as red pepper. Allicin itself, the pungent principle in garlic, is also toxic at very high doses, beyond what would ever be consumed by people. In animal studies, liver and stomach toxicity occurred after giving allicin to rats at a dose equivalent to a man eating 500 cloves of garlic. Allicin or fresh garlic can cause a minor side effect, because of its pungency, if it is held on the skin or the delicate tissues of the mouth, when it can cause irritation or actual burning. In some people who are sensitive, handling a lot of garlic can cause skin rashes; this is something that occasionally bothers professional cooks or workers in the food industry, who come in contact with garlic daily.

Since garlic can slow clotting, which is normally desirable for cardiovascular health, people who are taking anticlotting drugs should be aware that garlic can further reduce the clotting tendency of the blood. This could be a problem in certain situations, such as surgery. So, don't take a lot of garlic just before surgery.

In summary, there is no chance of any significant side effects of garlic at normal doses, whether fresh, dried, in the form of oil, or deodorized. The worst that can happen is that there may be some burping or mild stomach discomfort, if a lot of fresh garlic is eaten. This passes away after a few minutes. The smell is probably the only unwanted effect; it cannot properly be called a side effect, or one would have to say the same about the bad taste of penicillin. We have already discussed how the odor is removed in most garlic products.

There has been a good deal of controversy in the marketplace in recent years about which product to take, and the advantages of different products. A great deal of pseudoscientific statements have been made in the popular press, so that in the end, the public must feel that one cannot take garlic without a Ph.D. in chemistry. In this chapter, I have tried to demonstrate that there are different ways of preparing garlic, but that fortunately, for cardiovascular activity, most garlic preparations would be suitable. But don't forget, as with all plant remedies, fresh is best—and cheapest.

CHAPTER 10

Conclusion

The last two decades have seen a considerable improvement in the awareness of health. I remember twenty years ago going from bakery to bakery in the north of England looking for a good whole wheat loaf. Processed foods were the norm and anyone concerned about harmful food additives was regarded as an eccentric. The first vegetarian restaurant in London was deliberately named Cranks, as a play on the public image of vegetarians as sentimental faddists. Today, however, a great number of people know about the additives that are used in foods. Manufacturers are vying with each other to put "natural" on their labels, even if this is a questionable description of the contents. You can now buy health food and even organically grown foods in many supermarkets, and cholesterol has become the word for a household demon.

A LONG WAY TO GO

For all that, we have a very long way to go. In the United States, as in the United Kingdom and many other modern countries, the food industry lobby, the dairy lobby, the meat lobby, and the agricultural lobby have been very strong since the Second World War. Efforts to simplify and clean up the diet have not got very far. The official guidelines on healthy eating are pitifully conservative. We have already seen that the recommendation to scale back fat content from 40 percent to 30 percent of the diet will hardly have any effect on the plaque loading our blood vessels. A much more radical revision of our diet and lifestyle is needed—more on the lines of the Cretan or Japanese diets.

There is still a widespread assumption that heart disease is a misfortune that only affects some executives under stress, and that it is not worth worrying about unless your doctor tells you so. However, the doctor's function is curative, not preventive. Doctors have an extensive knowledge about what happens to the body if high blood pressure exists, and what drugs to use to depress it. But little is taught at medical school about how to prevent high blood pressure in the first place. That is left to the naturopaths, the health industry, and books and magazines, with some marginal help from the health education authorities. You cannot help but take your own health in hand and begin a program of self-care that is separate from and additional to anything your doctor might tell you.

Being more independent has its advantages and its risks. The advantage is that you learn more about yourself and your weaknesses and strengths. You can make a big difference, not only to your health, but also to your sense of well-being and control of your life. The disadvantage is that without the comforting medical authority, you may find yourself in a bewildering world of choices, fads, remedies, and promises, and it may be hard to find out what is right for you. However, your personal research will gradually untangle the principles behind the products, and from them, you can build your own health practices.

Modern medical treatments for cardiovascular disease usually come too little, too late. Strokes are considered to be more or less unpreventable. Heart bypass operations, when coolly evaluated, have been shown to extend the life span only marginally, and only in severe cases, since the new vessels soon develop plaque like the old ones. Cardiac intensive care can indeed save lives, but often home treatment in a less stressed environment, using holistic medicine, might have prevented the attack in the first place, and even afterwards might be as effective in stimulating recovery as the high-tech option. Cardiovascular drugs introduce a range of side effects that restrict the possible benefits. The message is clear: there are no panaceas in modern medicine. There is no choice but your path to prevention.

One question that is frequently asked is, why it is that remedies like garlic, and some of the other ideas presented in this book, are not already accepted by the establishment? One of the reasons is political, as I mentioned before, and has more to do with industrial lobbies than with health issues. Another reason is the nature of science and medical research. It is the pattern of the scientific culture that a therapeutic insight is true only if it can be demonstrated objectively by research studies. This puts very severe restrictions on what counts as fact. For example, it restricts the legitimacy of subjective experiences of illness or health, it restricts interest in more subtle methods of prevention and health maintenance, and it disallows states of health that do not have obvious symptoms, such as the buildup of fatty plaques in its early stages. For these reasons, it is often stated by the medical authorities that there is insufficient evidence to make more radical naturopathic recommendations to the public. This is a questionable argument.

Even after hundreds of millions of dollars spent on research, it is said that the importance of lowering cholesterol is still not established. Yet countries like Finland, which have launched serious preventive programs regardless, have lowered their levels of heart disease dramatically. We cannot wait for interminable research projects. Prevention should start now. Research can, and will, confirm it later.

GARLIC'S POPULARITY

Against this background, garlic has been one of the rediscoveries of the age. It has been taken in large quantities for many years to aid coughs, colds, catarrh, sore throats, and other persistent infections. Now it is being brought into the limelight through its ability to help diseases of the circulatory system. There is so much evidence of its effects that it is becoming one of the most popular remedies in the modern world.

Garlic is the people's medicine. It is not a rare or special remedy, nor a pure drug with a patent on it, nor an expensive pharmaceutical concoction. Like all our herbal remedies and medicinal foods, it is part of our inheritance. With the growing movement towards herbs and natural remedies, pharmacies are looking more and more like health shops, and health shops are becoming a little like pharmacies. In France and Germany especially, pharmacies now have a distinctly herbaceous atmosphere, more so than at any time since the days of the apothecaries. Garlic naturally has an important place in this new movement.

The herbal tradition itself has gone through a major transition in the last few years, accompanying its rise in popularity. It is no longer full of old-fashioned, musty-smelling, peculiar remedies. Today, herbalism is called *phytotherapy,* and its herbs are often concentrated extracts prepared under scientifically controlled conditions, and analyzed in the laboratory to ensure purity and sufficient concentrations of the active constituents. Herbs come in tablets and capsules, licensed by health authorities in a similar manner to pharmaceuticals. Garlic is a part of this revolution. As its popularity has increased, so has our knowledge of its effects and how to prepare and process it. We are beginning to benefit both from the experience of the past and from the modern research programs.

GARLIC AND THE MEDICAL ESTABLISHMENT

Garlic is still not yet fully recognized by the medical establishments of all countries. In this respect, it is held back by the regulatory attitude to herbs as a whole, which are not given special status under the law, but treated in the same way as synthetic pharmaceutical drugs. Although at least thirty clinical trials were published during the last ten years, almost all on the cardiovascular effects of garlic, they were sufficient only to convince the health authorities in Germany, where most of them were carried out. There have been a couple of serious clinical studies in the United States, but until more trials are carried out, and there is major pharmaceutical backing for garlic, the FDA is unlikely to accept it fully or license it. Although garlic oil has a license from the authorities in the United Kingdom, this only allows manufacturers of garlic products to make claims of its effectiveness in relation to coughs, catarrh, and other such illnesses. This does not mean that garlic oil does not work as a cardiovascular preventive in Britain, only that the British health authorities are not yet convinced of it! They have not yet caught up with our full knowledge of garlic's effects. Only in Germany and one or two other European countries is garlic acknowledged by the authorities to be an effective preventive remedy for circulation problems.

Nevertheless, it is likely that we will now see accelerated research programs designed to find out exactly how strong garlic is as a cardiovascular disease preventative, and how it compares with modern chemical drugs on the one hand and with other natural medicinal preparations such as EPA-rich fish oil on the other. We still do not really know how strong it is and what kinds of people will benefit most from it. There is also a need for more research on its anti-infective effects on humans, which would complement that research already done in the laboratory.

THE TRUE PLACE OF NATURAL REMEDIES

For most of this century, we have been used to drugs. These are single chemical compounds with an exact and known action on a body process. They are strong and specific; their side effects arise because their action on one particular part of the body can unleash unexpected changes elsewhere. These drugs replaced the herbs that were the mainstay of medicine before them. Herbs were deposed because they were regarded as unscientific, unreliable, weak, and messy. Now that we know the problems drugs can cause, there is a renewal of interest in herbal remedies. We find that most of them were removed from the pharmacopoeias without any rational justification. They were not dismissed because they were useless, since their effectiveness had not been tested in the laboratory. They were dismissed for the very unscientific reason that they didn't fit into the system.

Now that herbs are returning to our medicine chest, we should ask ourselves whether or not the original criticisms were true. They turn out to have been true only from the medical perspective that diagnoses a precise set of symptoms and then uses specific drugs to eradicate them. A more traditional, natural, or "complementary" approach is to reduce the vulnerability or susceptibility to the disease and encourage the body to overcome it by itself. Herbs fit very well into this approach. They often have effects that are adjustive—that is, effects that work with the body rather than against it. For example, herbs like echinacea, yarrow, or licorice can support and encourage the body's immunity and help it throw off an infection. No present-day drug is able to achieve such an effect. Garlic, likewise, is able to prevent diseases of the circulation in a way unmatched by any modern medicine. Common herbs such as mint, comfrey, coltsfoot, feverfew, and thousands of others can deal with symptoms without upsetting the built-in natural healing process.

Herbs are, it is true, weaker than pure chemicals and do not dispose of symptoms so fast. However, they are more gentle and keep closer to the original medical maxim, "First, do no harm." Their weakness can be a disadvantage if you have a serious, runaway infection. On the other hand, an herb can affect a range of processes that otherwise would require a whole battery of drugs. We have seen this in the cardiovascular system, where garlic affects blood clotting, blood pressure, cholesterol, and thinness of the blood, as well as its other useful effects, such as getting rid of extra body water.

These properties make herbs irreplaceable in prevention and in the self-treatment of many minor or chronic problems. Whether or not you wish to use them for more serious conditions will depend to a large extent on professional advice. Herbs can be used for virtually all health problems, either alone or with other forms of treatment. However, expert advice will enable you to get the best from them, and this should always be sought when dealing with serious illnesses.

THE LIMITS OF SELF-CARE

Three-quarters of all health problems never arrive in the doctor's waiting room. Most of them are mild and self-limiting—that is, they pass away by themselves, and are dealt with in daily life. For every episode of chest pain that is caused by angina, there will be thousands that are due to a passing tightness in the muscles, or intestinal gas pressing on the diaphragm, and therefore nothing to worry about or to treat medically.

In other words, people mostly look after themselves. Mild remedies like garlic or other herbs or vitamins are helpful in this because they provide the tools of self-care. However, their true effectiveness depends on how much you know. The more you know about garlic, for example, the less you will find yourself at the doctor's office asking for an antibiotic. In the modern world a great deal of this knowledge has been lost. We have been encouraged to take all our problems to the expert, who will deal with them without even telling us what he is doing. Indeed, given the strength of modern drugs, it is a good thing that we do not treat ourselves with them. But because of this general lack of knowledge, we start at a disadvantage. The only way to overcome this is to learn. That is why so many health books are written and read. It is a process of relearning about the natural medicines all around us.

Nevertheless, for the proper treatment of any medical condition by herbs and diet, you would be well advised to seek professional advice. This does not mean that you cannot help yourself; it means that you might achieve better results if your efforts were monitored and guided by a health professional. In the case of the heart and circulatory system, it would be as well to have occasional checkups. If everything is satisfactory, then you do not need professional help in treatment. However, you may still appreciate some advice on a regimen of general health maintenance to suit your personal situation. If your professional advisor finds that you are potentially vulnerable to cardiovascular problems, he may be able to design a regimen that will be more effective than your own. For example, he may recommend certain herbs to take along with garlic, or he may review your diet with you. The professionals who are best able to work with you in this way are naturopaths, herbalists, and many homoeopaths or holistic doctors. Conventional doctors who do not have a holistic training are not so adept, but with the rise of complementary medicine there are more experts able to assist your efforts.

There remains the question of how one should take in and use all the information now available on health care. This is the second book I have written on garlic, and each time, people have asked me how it is possible to write a whole book on the subject. I reply, quoting William Blake, that it is possible to see a world in a grain of sand. However, as far as health is concerned, there is so much advice and information today, in the form of thousands of books, articles, and other materials, that it is not possible for everyone to be an expert on all the regimens, remedies, and supplements. From the books and information, as I mentioned, you can glean some basic principles of self-care, and also some particular remedies that might feel right for you. But there is another process that is as important as any health advice. It is to start researching the inner context as well as the outer one. Concentrate on learning about yourself, noticing your body, and observing your general condition, just like the careful car owner who knows how to listen to his engine and always seems to have his vehicle on the road when all the rest have broken down. Then it will become clear to you which are the essential self-care tools you need. With its wide applicability, long tradition of reliable use, and great safety, garlic will surely be one of them.

Further Reading

Books on Garlic

Fulder, S. and Blackwood, J. *Garlic, Nature's Original Remedy.* Rochester, VT: Healing Arts Press, 1993.

Koch, H.P. and Lawson, L.D. *Garlic—The Science and Therapeutic Application of* Allium Sativum L. *and Related Species.* Baltimore, MD: Williams and Wilkins, 1996.

Selected Scientific References

Garlic Chemistry

Block, E. "The Chemistry of Garlic and Onions." *Scientific American*, 252, 94–97, 1985.

Brodnitz, M.H. et al. "Flavor Components of Garlic Extract." *Journal of Agricultural Food Chemistry*, 19, 273–275, 1971.

Fenwick, G.R. and Hanley, A.B. "The Genus Allium," Parts 1–3, *Critical Reviews on Food Science*, Vols 22 and 23, 199–271 and 273–377, 1986.

Lawson, L.D. and Hughes, B. "Characterization of the

Formation of Allicin and Other Thiosulfinates from Garlic." *Planta Medica*, 58, 345–350, 1992.

Lawson, L.D. "Bioactive Organosulfur Compounds of Garlic and Garlic Products: Role in Reducing Blood Lipids." In *Human Medicinal Agents from Plants* (Kinghorn, A.D. and Balandrin, M.F., eds). Washington, D.C.: American Chemical Society Books, 1993.

Garlic's Effects on the Circulation

Apitz-Castro, R. et al. "Ajoene, the Antiplatelet Principle of Garlic." *Thrombosis Research*, 42, 303–311, 1986.

Banerjee, A.K. "Effect of Aqueous Extract of Garlic on Arterial Blood Pressure of Normotensive and Hypertensive Rats." *Artery*, 2, 369–373, 1976.

Bordia, A. et al. "Effects of the Essential Oils of Garlic and Onion on Alimentary Hyperlipidaemia." *Atherosclerosis*, 21, 15–19, 1975.

Bordia, A. and Verma, S.K. "Effect of Garlic Feeding on Regression of Experimental Atherosclerosis in Rabbits." *Artery*, 7, 428–437, 1980.

Bordia, A. "Effect of Garlic on Blood Lipids in Patients with Coronary Heart Disease." *American Journal of Clinical Nutrition*, 34, 200–203, 1981.

Boullin, D.J. "Garlic as a Platelet Inhibitor." *Lancet*, 1, 776–777, 1981.

Chi, M.S. et al. "Effects of Garlic on Lipid Metabolism in Rats Fed Cholesterol or Lard." *Journal of Nutrition*, 112, 41–48, 1982.

Chutani, S.K. and Bordia, A. "The Effect of Fried Versus Raw Garlic on Fibrinolytic Activity in Man." *Atherosclerosis*, 38, 417–421, 1981.

De A Santos, O.S. and Grunwald, J. "Effect of Garlic Powder Tablets on Blood Lipids and Blood Pressure: a Six Month, Placebo Controlled, Double-Blind Study." *British Journal of Clinical Research*, 4, 37–44, 1993.

De Boer, L.W.V. and Folts, J.D. "Garlic Extract Prevents Acute Platelet Thrombus Formation in Stenosed Canine Coronary Arteries." *American Heart Journal*, 117, 973–975, 1989.

Ernst, E. et al. "Garlic and Blood Lipids." *British Medical Journal*, 291, 139, 1985.

Editorial, "Natural Fibrinolysis and its Stimulation." *Lancet*, 1, 1401–1402, 1982.

Foushee, D.B. et al. "Garlic as a Natural Agent for the Treatment of Hypertension: a Preliminary Report." *Cytobios*, 34, 145–152, 1982.

Jain, A.K., Vargas, R., Gotzkowsky, S. and MacMahon, F.G. "Can Garlic Reduce Levels of Serum Lipids? A Controlled Clinical Study." *American Journal of Medicine*, 94, 632–635, 1993.

Jung, F., Jung, E.M., Pindur, G. and Kieswetter, H. "Effect of Different Garlic Preparations on the Fluidity of Blood, Fibrinolytic Activity, and Peripheral Microcirculation in Comparison with Placebo." *Planta Medica*, 56, 668, 1990.

Keyes, A. "Wine, Garlic, and CHD in Seven Countries." *Lancet*, 145–146, 1980.

Mader, F.H. "Treatment of Hyperlipidaemia with Garlic-powder Tablets." *Drug Research*, 40, 1111–1116, 1990.

Makheja, A.N. et al. "Inhibition of Platelet Aggregation and Thromboxane Synthesis by Onion and Garlic." *Lancet*, 781, 1979.

Sainani, B.S. et al. "Effect of Dietary Garlic and Onion on Serum Lipid Profile in a Jain Community." *Indian Journal of Medical Research*, 69, 776–780, 1979.

Silagy, C. and Neil, A. "Garlic as a Lipid-Lowering Agent: a Meta-Analysis." *Journal of the Royal College of Physicians*, 28, 39–45, 1994.

Srivastava, K.C. "Evidence for the Mechanism by Which Garlic Inhibits Platelet Aggregation." *Prostaglandins Leukotrene Medicine*, 22, 313–321, 1986.

Warshafsky, S., Kamer, R.S. and Sivak, S.L. "Effect of Garlic on Total Serum Cholesterol: a Meta-Analysis." *Annals of Internal Medicine*, 119, 599–605, 1993.

Garlic Against Infections

Adetumbi, M.A. and Lau, B.H.S. "Allium sativum (garlic)—A Natural Antibiotic." *Medical Hypotheses*, 12, 227–237, 1983.

Amer, M. et al. "The Effect of Aqueous Garlic Extract on the Growth of Dermatophytes." *International Journal of Dermatology*, 19, 285–287, 1980.

Caporaso, L. et al. "Antifungal Activity in Human Urine and Serum After Ingestion of Garlic *(Allium sativum)*." *Antimicrobial Agents and Chemotherapy*, 23, 700–702, 1983.

Davis, L.E. et al. "Antifungal Activity in Human Cerebrospinal Fluid and Plasma after Intravenous Administration of *Allium sativum*." *Antimicrobial Agents and Chemotherapy*, 34, 651–653, 1990.

Hughes, B. G. and Lawson, L.D. "Antimicrobial Effects of *Allium sativum L.* (garlic), *Allium ampeloprasum* (elephant garlic), and *Allium cepa* (onion), Garlic Compounds and

Commercial Garlic Supplement Products." *Phytotherapy Research*, 5, 154–158, 1991.

Mirelman, D. et al. "Inhibition of Growth of Entamoeba Histolytica by Allicin, the Active Principle of Garlic Extract." *Journal of Infectious Diseases*, 156, 243–244, 1987.

Moore, G.S. and Atkins, R.D. "Fungicidal and Fungistatic Effects of an Aqueous Garlic Extract on Medically Important Yeast-Like Fungi." *Mycologia*, 69, 341–348, 1997.

Rees, L.P. et al. "A Quantitative Assessment of the Antimicrobial Activity of Garlic *(Allium sativum)*." *World Journal of Microbiology and Biotechnology*, 9, 303–307, 1993.

Shoji, S. et al. "Allyl Compounds Selectively Killed Human Immunodeficiency Virus (type 1)—infected Cells." *Biochemical Biophysics Research Communication*, 194, 610–621.

Warner, J. "Garlic Wards Off Undead Bacteria." *New Scientist*, No. 5, 17, 1994.

Garlic and Blood Sugar

Augusti, K.T. "Studies on the Effect of Allicin (diallyl-disulphide-oxide) on Alloxan Diabetes." *Experientia*, 31, 1263–1265, 1975.

Chang, M.L.W. and Johnson, M.A. "Effect of Garlic on Carbohydrate Metabolism and Lipid Synthesis in Rats." *Journal of Nutrition*, 110, 931–936, 1980.

Jain, R.C. et al. "Hypoglycaemic Action of Onion and Garlic." *Lancet*, 1491, 1973.

Garlic, Tumor Prevention, and Antitoxicity

Belman, S. "Onion and Garlic Oils and Tumor Promotion." *Carcinogenesis*, 4, 1063–1065, 1983.

Dorant, E. et al. "Garlic and its Significance in the Prevention of Cancer in Humans, a Critical Review," *British Journal of Cancer*, 67, 424–429, 1993.

Han, J. "Highlights of the Cancer Chemoprevention Studies in China." *Preventive Medicine*, 22, 712–722, 1993.

Roychoudhury, A. et al. "Use of Crude Extracts of Garlic *(Allium sativum L.)* in Reducing Cytotoxic Effects of Arsenic in Mouse Bone Marrow." *Phytotherapy Research*, 7, 163–166, 1993.

Steinmetz, K.A. et al. "Vegetables, Fruit, and Colon Cancer in the Iowa Women's Health Study." *American Journal of Epidemiology*, 139, 1–15, 1994.

Sundaraman, S.G. and Milner, J.A. "Diallyl Disulfide in Garlic Oil Inhibits Both *in vitro* and *in vivo* Growth of Human Colon Tumor Cells." *FASEB Journal*, 9, A869, 1995.

Wargovich, M.J. "Diallyl Sulphide, a Flavor Component of Garlic (Allium sativum), Inhibits Dimethylhydrazine Induced Colon Cancer." *Carcinogenesis*, 8, 487–489, 1987.

Wargovich, M.J. "Inhibition of Gastrointestinal Cancer by Organosulfur Compounds in Garlic." *Cancer Chemoprevention*, 195–203, 1992.

Weisberger, H.S. and Pensky, J. "Tumor-Inhibiting Effects Derived from an Active Principle of Garlic (*Allium sativum*)." *Science*, 126, 1112–1114, 1957.

Index